Materia Medica for Nurses

Materia Medica
for Nurses
A Textbook of Drugs and Therapeutics

W. GORDON SEARS

M.D. (Lond.), M.R.C.P. (Lond.)
HONORARY CONSULTANT PHYSICIAN, MILE END HOSPITAL, LONDON

AND

R. S. WINWOOD

M.B., M.R.C.P.
CONSULTANT PHYSICIAN, WHIPPS CROSS HOSPITAL, LONDON

SEVENTH EDITION

 London EDWARD ARNOLD (Publishers) Ltd

© W. GORDON SEARS
AND R. S. WINWOOD 1971

First Published	1943
by Edward Arnold (Publishers) Ltd.,	
41 Maddox Street, London, WIR OAN	
Reprinted	1943, 1944 (*twice*), 1945
Second Edition	1947
Reprinted	1948
Third Edition	1955
Reprinted	1958
Fourth Edition	1959
Fifth Edition	1962
Reprinted	1964
Sixth Edition	1966
Reprinted	1968
Seventh Edition	1971

ISBN: Boards 0 7131 4189 1

Paper 0 7131 4190 5

Printed in Great Britain by
C. Tinling & Co. Ltd. London and Prescot

Preface to the Seventh Edition

It will be generally agreed that the compilation of a modern work on the subject of drugs, at any level, is no easy problem to solve for many reasons:—

1. Old remedies and placebos die hard and may still be used.
2. Many new drugs come into use every year, and to attempt to include all the drugs that a nurse may encounter would be impossible.
3. Their chemical constitution, the complexity of their names and pharmacological action is clearly often beyond the scope of the basic training and memory of most nurses and many doctors.

As far as possible both Official and the more common proprietary names are given (the latter in inverted commas). Likewise in addition to metric doses, Imperial measures are included when these may be helpful to some.

We are very grateful to Mrs E. M. Fell, M.P.S., Deputy Chief Pharmacist at the Norfolk and Norwich Hospital who helped with the section on the D.D.A.

Dr R. S. Winwood has, after most helpful co-operation in the preparation of the last Edition, now joined in the authorship of this book as he has done in the recent new edition of "Medicine for Nurses".

London, 1971   W. GORDON SEARS

From the Preface to the Seventh Edition

Nurses are constantly handling drugs to which they can find no reference in their ordinary text-books, and a spirit of enquiry is so often manifest, as Tutors and Ward Sisters will know, that I have not hesitated to include as many drugs as possible in the space at my disposal.

Materia Medica in its old-fashioned sense which deals with the various vegetable preparations and their botanical origin is of little importance to the nurse. On the other hand, the modern confusion of proprietary preparations, with and without official names, is a most difficult subject to comprehend, but at the same time is extremely important. Many of the more familiar proprietary preparations have, therefore, been mentioned.

Some stress has been laid on therapeutic procedures, signs of over-dosage and points which the nurse can observe or has to carry out for herself.

I would emphasize that this work, like my others, is not intended to be just put into a nurse's hands for her to learn the subject for an examination. The intention is that she should learn from it what it is necessary for her to know under the guidance of a competent teacher, for a nurse in training requires a teacher to indicate:

1. What she should learn for her examinations.
2. What she should read for her own interest.
3. What is included merely for reference.

With this in view, small print has been used for matter which may definitely be included in the last category. In attempting to combine these three factors, a somewhat larger book than is usual for nurses has resulted. However, this has not been used as an excuse to produce an expensive work, and every effort has been made to keep its cost as low as possible.

Contents

CHAPTER 1

Introduction

The subject of Drugs and their uses is a very large one and has many branches. It is constantly expanding and, while new drugs are being discovered, others are falling into disuse.

DEFINITIONS

1. The term **Materia Medica** may be used to include the whole subject.

2. A **Drug** is any substance taken into the body or applied to its surface for the prevention or treatment of disease.

3. **Pharmacy** is the art of preparing drugs in the various forms suitable for their administration, such as tinctures and extracts. Included in pharmacy is the practice of **Dispensing** which involves the compounding of preparations such as pills, mixtures and ointments from their various constituents. However so many therapeutic substances are now mass-produced that the modern pharmacist is mainly responsible for their care and distribution.

4. **Pharmacology** deals with the mode of action of various drugs. It endeavours to explain on which organs of the body a drug acts and exactly how it operates. It is, therefore, closely united with physiology. For example, pharmacology explains how digitalis acts on the bundle of His in the heart, slows the rate of the ventricle in atrial fibrillation and improves the strength of cardiac contraction.

Drugs given in excessive amounts are liable to act as poisons, the study of which is called **Toxicology.**

5. **Therapeutics** is the art of using remedies in the treatment of disease. It embraces all the methods employed in the management and care of a patient whereby we endeavour to aid Nature in restoring the individual to health. Included also are the efforts made to relieve the patient's symptoms even if the disease cannot

be cured, i.e. remedies may be (*a*) symptomatic, (*b*) palliative or (*c*) curative.

The British Pharmacopoeia

The British Pharmacopoeia (B.P.) is a list of "official" drugs and their doses published by the General Medical Council. It lays down the chemical standard which must be maintained in the manufacture of all drugs labelled 'B.P.' and is revised from time to time.

The British Pharmaceutical Codex (B.P.C.) is an "unofficial" work published by the Pharmaceutical Society of Great Britain which acts as a supplement to the B.P. and contains a number of other drugs and useful preparations.

The British National Formulary (B.N.F.) is a handbook which includes those drugs and preparations in common use, and is widely employed both in hospital and general practice as a basis for prescribing. There are also many useful notes on drugs which a nurse may well study.

Proprietary preparations. In addition to the official and semiofficial preparations, there are an enormous number of drugs prepared and sold by firms of manufacturing chemists all over the world. Some of them are very valuable, others are more or less useless, but it is only fair to say that many advances in therapeutics and the introduction of useful new drug are due to the research and enterprise of these commercial undertakings. A number of these preparations ultimately become "official" and are included in the B.P., usually under a different name.

This is often very confusing because a drug is known for some years by its proprietary name and only later does the "official" or "approved" term come into general use For example, phenobarbitone became the "official" name for "Luminal". Most of the proprietary preparations in use are listed in such publications as MIMS.

(N.B.—Proprietary names are denoted in the present text in inverted commas.)

TERMINOLOGY

One of the most difficult and confusing aspects of the subject to the beginner is the terminology used in the naming of drugs. In the first place it must be understood that therapeutic substances are of very varied origin.

1. Vegetable

Drugs may be obtained from various parts of many plants such as their leaves, roots, seeds, flowers, fruit or bark. Resins and some oils are also obtained from vegetable sources.

The modern tendency has been to extract the active principles from medicinal plants rather than to use the actual plants. There are, however, some exceptions to this rule, e.g. (*a*) The use of senna pods to make the laxative, senna tea. (*b*) The use of powdered digitalis leaves (*Digitalis folia*) in the treatment of heart disease.

The two most important types of active principles extracted are:

(*a*) Alkaloids.
(*b*) Glycosides.

Alkaloids. These are usually highly active substances which are only used in very small doses. They contain nitrogen and their names generally terminate in -INE (*in Latin -ina*) thus:

> Morphine is an alkaloid of opium.
> Strychnine   „   „   „ nux vomica.
> Atropine   „   „   „ belladonna.
> Nicotine   „   „   „ tobacco.

Glycosides or **glucosides.** These are very potent vegetable substances in the formation of which glucose, or some other sugar, takes part.

> Digoxin is a glycoside of digitalis.

The names of the glycosides terminate in -IN, although not every substance ending in this way is a glycoside, e.g. liquid paraffin is a mineral oil.

2. Mineral

This group includes well-known natural substances such as iron, bismuth, mercury and common chemical compounds like Epsom salts (magnesium sulphate), Glauber's salt (sodium sulphate) and various compounds of lime (calcium) and phosphorus (phosphates).

3. Animal

This term applies in particular to vaccines, sera, gland extracts, hormones and similar preparations.

4. Synthetic

The term "synthetic" is used to describe a large number of drugs, some of them very complicated in composition, which are prepared in chemical laboratories (e.g. the sulphonamides). The composition of many natural substances is also known, and some can be prepared chemically as well as being obtained from their natural sources. For example, adrenaline can be obtained from the suprarenal gland, but is more economically manufactured by ordinary chemical processes.

5. Antibiotics

These drugs play a very important part in the modern treatment of infections and consist of antibacterial substances derived from various moulds. They may be defined as chemical substances produced by micro-organisms, which prevent the growth of other micro-organisms. Some of these can now be made synthetically. The best known examples are penicillin, streptomycin, the tetracyclines and chloramphenicol (p. 231).

CLASSIFICATION OF DRUGS

It is convenient in a text-book to consider drugs acting on the various systems of the body together. It is also useful to classify them in general terms which indicate their main action. Although individual drugs will be dealt with in appropriate chapters the following definitions in common use may be found helpful.

Analgesics and anodyne drugs are used to relieve pain.

Antacids neutralize hydrochloric acid in the stomach.

Anthelmintics are used in the treatment of intestinal worms.

Anticoagulants such as heparin and 'Dindevan' diminish the clotting power of the blood.

Anticonvulsants are used in the treatment of epilepsy and other states in which irritation of the brain results in fits or convulsions; e.g. phenobarbitone.

Antidepressants stimulate the higher centres of the brain. They may cause wakefulness and a temporary feeling of well-being; e.g. amphetamine.

Antidiabetic drugs. In addition to insulin, the oral hypoglycaemic agents tolbutamide and chlorpropamide ('Diabinese') lower the blood sugar in diabetes.

Antihistamines counteract the action of histamine, a substance liberated in the tissues in a number of allergic conditions such as hay fever and urticaria.

Antipruritics are drugs which relieve itching.

Diuretics increase the secretion of urine.

Haemopoietic drugs stimulate the formation of red cells, e.g. vitamin B_{12} in the treatment of pernicious anaemia.

Haematinics contain iron necessary for the formation of haemoglobin.

Haemostatics stop bleeding and help in the clotting of blood.

Hypnotics help in the production of sleep.

Sedatives and tranquillizers help to calm the nervous system.

Thymoleptic drugs help to change the mood of the patient in states of depression and anxiety (see p. 150).

In Great Britain the use of Latin names for drugs is no longer recommended and their English titles should be used in prescribing. Likewise, the Metric System has replaced the Apothecary's and the Imperial measures.

Many of the synthetic drugs are extremely complicated chemical compounds with very long names, the meaning of which is only appreciated by a chemist. In such instances, simpler names are often given, either "officially" or as a trade name by the manufacturer. As a rule the "official" name differs from the trade name as the latter is protected by Law and may only be used by the manufacturer. For example, Aspirin was the trade name for acetylsalicylic acid which was originally owned by Bayer. 'Chloromycetin' is a trade name for chloramphenicol, 'Epanutin' is the trade name of phenytoin.

THE LEGAL CONTROL OF DRUGS

Because many drugs are very powerful poisons if employed in improper doses, and others have dangerous habit-forming properties (see p. 147), the manufacture, distribution and care of a number of such drugs are carefully protected by Law.

There are two Acts which deal with drugs:
1. The Dangerous Drugs Act (D.D.A.).
2. The Poisons Act.

(These Acts are supplemented by the Dangerous Drugs Regulations and Poisons Regulations made in connection with the respective Acts.)

Certain details of these Acts and Regulations are of importance to the nurse.

The Dangerous Drugs Act (D.D.A.)

The object of this Act is to prevent the improper sale of drugs having dangerous habit-forming properties. Under it the following important drugs and most of their preparations are controlled:

Opium.

Morphine. Papaveretum ('Omnopon'). 'Nepenthe'.

Pethidine, 'Pethilorfan'. Methadone ('Amidone', 'Physeptone', including *Linctus*).

Levorphanol ('Dromoran'). 'Proladone'. 'Diconal'.

Cocaine.

Diamorphine. (Heroin), including Diamorphine linctus.

N.B.—Heroin can only be manufactured under special licence. Its importation into many countries is forbidden on account of its liability to produce addiction.

Indian hemp (*Cannabis satira*) (see p. 150).

Certain preparations containing only small amounts of the above drugs are exempt from the D.D.A., but nevertheless are controlled by the 'Poisons' Act—e.g.:

'Dover's powder' (*Pulvis ipecacuanhae et opii*).

'Chlorodyne' (*Tinct. Chloroformi et Morphini Co.*).

Among rules governing the handling of these drugs are:

1. They can only be ordered by a doctor.

2. In private practice the doctor must keep a record of all purchases and supplies in a separate register or part of a register for each drug.

He must record the amount of the drug actually issued to patients, but is not bound to record the drugs actually administered to patients by himself or under his personal supervision in his presence.

3. Special rules are applied in hospitals, and although the details may vary in different institutions, certain general principles which must fulfil the law are applicable to all.

(*a*) All drugs controlled by the Act must be kept in a special poison cupboard (which should be marked D.D.A.). This cupboard must be kept locked and the key retained *on the person of* the nurse in charge of the ward or department, usually a State Registered Nurse, who is entirely responsible for the safe custody of the drugs.

(*b*) Fresh supplies can only be obtained from the Pharmacist on an order signed by a Medical Officer or the nurse in charge of the ward. The drugs should be checked on arrival by the nurse in charge of the ward and the form of written receipt given.

(c) A register should be kept with separate sections for each drug. Every dose administered must be recorded together with the date, name of the patient and the amount given. This should be filled in and signed by the person giving the drug.

(d) These drugs may only be given on the written instructions of a doctor.

It is advisable also that the following details be carried out, although they do not form part of the actual regulations:

(a) Each dose given should be checked by an independent witness who sees the phial from which the drug is taken together with the written order of the doctor.

(b) The hospital Pharmacist should inspect and check the dangerous drugs in the wards and compare the stocks with the entries in the Dangerous Drugs Register at regular intervals.

(c) All bottles should be marked with a red D.D.A. label.

(d) Sometimes the supply of a dangerous drug, which is not normally part of the ward stock, is ordered for one patient. For example, morphine suppositories, diamorphine linctus or a special mixture containing one of these drugs. In such instances, if the whole supply is not used, the correct procedure is for the nurse in charge to return the surplus personally to the Pharmacist.

Poisons Act and Rules

In addition to the D.D.A., the care and distribution of a large number of other substances are controlled by law.

There can be no standard definition of a poison because, clearly, the poisonous effect of any substance depends on the dose given. However, for legal purposes a certain arbitrary standard has been selected and the most dangerous substances are called "Poisons" and are included in the "Poisons List". Not all these substances are necessarily used in medicine but in order that the Regulations can be carried out according to Law they are also classified into a number of Schedules. Schedules 1 and 4 are mainly applicable in hospital work.

The Regulations and rules associated with these substances not only concern their sale to members of the public but also to their storage, issue to hospital patients and the methods by which they are labelled.

Schedule 1 (which includes D.D.A.)

The rules state that any of these drugs which are kept in the

wards of a hospital must be stored in a cupboard reserved solely
for poisons and other dangerous substances. (N.B.—Special
additional rules apply to D.D.A. drugs.)

Schedule 4

For purposes of storage and labelling in hospital this schedule
is now divided into the groups 4A and 4B. All drugs in Schedule 4A
are included in Schedule 1 and the following rules apply:

The *general public* can only obtain the drugs listed in Schedule 4
on the production of a medical prescription signed by a doctor.

In hospitals. (i) These drugs are only supplied to wards from
the dispensary on the written order of a Medical Officer or the
nurse in charge of the ward.

(ii) The container of the substance must be labelled with the
name of its contents and the more powerful poisons (listed in
Schedule 1) bear a distinguishing label to indicate that they
must be kept in a poison cupboard, specially reserved for such
drugs.

(iii) Poison cupboards should be kept locked and must be
inspected by the Pharmacist at regular intervals.

(iv) Drugs for internal administration which are listed in the
poison Schedules should be kept separate from preparations
intended for external use.

Out-patients. (i) These drugs are only supplied on the written
order of the doctor.

(ii) A record of the issue must be kept for two years on a case
paper or card stating the name and address of the patient, the
name or initials of the prescriber, the date and amount of the
poison supplied.

(iii) The container must be labelled with the name of the hospital
supplying it. If it is a lotion, liniment or other medicament for
external application, it must be marked "The Liniment" (or
appropriate title), "For external use only".

Special poison bottles of characteristic shape which can be
recognized by touch (e.g. having vertical ridges and grooves)
must be used.

Schedule 4B

These drugs are not listed in Schedule 1 and are not subject to
the special stringent regulations applicable to this schedule. They
must, however, be labelled "Poison" or "Caution" such as "It is

dangerous to exceed the stated dose", but they may be stored with other medicines if necessary.

The D.D.A. and Schedule drugs are appropriately noted in the National Formulary and only a few examples are given.

Schedule 1
In addition to the drugs controlled by the D.D.A., most alkaloids and other powerful poisons (except in certain specified weak dilutions) are included, e.g.

Aconite	
Apomorphine	Barbiturates
Atropine and belladonna	Carbachol
Codeine, 'DF 118'	Digitalis preparations
Curare	Some mercury preparations
Emetine	Mersalyl, 'Neptal'
Ergot alkaloids	Nalorphine
Hyoscine and hyoscyamine	Nitrogen mustard and other
Strychnine and nux vomica	cytotoxic drugs

Schedule 4A
As already mentioned all the drugs in this list are included in Schedule 1, e.g.

Barbiturates and preparations containing them
Mercaptopurine

Schedule 4B
This schedule covers the sulphonamides, tranquillizers, oestrogens, amphetamine, chlorpromazine, methyl pentynol ('Oblivon'), reserpine, phenylbutazone, hypoglycaemic agents such as chlorpropamide ('Diabinese') and many other drugs.

CHAPTER 2

Pharmaceutical Preparations

There are a number of preparations in use some of which are only occasionally encountered. Those commonly employed are listed in the B.N.F.

Aerosols
e.g salbutamol ('Ventolin') aerosol for asthma.

Applications or applicationes

There are various preparations which are applied to the surface of the body:
e.g. Benzyl benzoate applications (*Applicatio benzylis benzoatis*).
Dicophane (DDT) application (*Applicatio dicophani*).

Cachets or capsulae amylaceae

These are composed of two discs made of rice flour, the edges of which adhere when moistened. The drug is placed between the discs before sealing. When the whole cachet is moistened it becomes soft and is easily swallowed, it is therefore especially useful for giving a powdered drug.
e.g. 'Pasinah—302' cachets.

Capsules or capsulae

These are containers usually made of gelatin. Cachets and capsules are generally used for unpleasant drugs and are intended to be swallowed like pills.
e.g. Vitamin capsules (*Capsulae vitaminorum*).
Quinalbarbitone capsules (*Capsulae quinalbarbitoni*),
Ampicillin capsules.
'Spansules' are special proprietary capsules designed to give a regulated, slow release of the drugs they contain.

Collodions or collodia

These are substances dissolved in a volatile and highly in-flammable solvent which evaporates when applied to the surface of the body, leaving a film-like skin or protective covering.

e.g. Flexible collodion (*Collodium flexile*).

    (i) **Eye lotions** or **collyria** (p. 12, 214).

    (ii) **Mouth washes** or **collutoria** (p. 59).

    (iii) **Nasal douches** or **collunaria** (p. 120).

Creams

Creams are similar to ointments but contain water and an emulsifying agent. Their ingredients are more penetrating and more easily absorbed than from greasy ointments.

e.g. Calamine cream (*Cremor calamini*).

    Zinc oxide cream (*Cremor zinci oxidi*).

Draughts or haustus

Drugs in mixture form which are intended to be administered as a single dose are often called draughts.

The administration of a single dose distinguishes them from mixtures, which are usually intended for repeated doses at regular intervals. e.g. Male fern extract draught.

Dusting-powders or conspersi

These are applied locally to the skin.

e.g. Talc dusting-powder (*Conspersus talci borici*).

    Dicophane (DDT) dusting-powder (*Conspersus dicophani*).

Ear-drops or auristillae

e.g. Phenol ear-drops (*Auristillae phenolis*) (p. 40).

Elixirs or elixiria

Elixirs are sweet liquid preparations containing syrup, glycerin and, sometimes, alcohol to which various drugs are added. They are very pleasant but rather expensive.

e.g. Elixir of cascara sagrada (*Elixir cascarae sagradae*).

Emulsions or emulsiones

There are many substances which will not normally mix together, such as oil and water, but which may be combined by the additon of a third substance called an emulsifying agent. In an emulsion the globules of fat or oil, instead of running together, remain separate. In some cases the oil and water tend to separate into layers on standing, in spite of the presence of an emulsifying agent, but will re-form an emulsion on shaking. Acacia gum and tragacanth are common emulsifying agents. Milk is an excellent example of a natural emulsion.

e.g. Liquid paraffin emulsion (*Emulsio paraffini liquidi*).

Enemas or enemata (p. 74).

Strictly speaking, an enema consists of the rectal injection of a small quantity of fluid and does not include the administration of large infusions of saline or glucose. Enemas may be classified in the following way:

1. *Those to be returned.*

   Aperient or evacuant: warm water, arachis oil, soap, glycerin, turpentine.

2. *Those to be retained.*

   Sedative: starch, starch and opium.

   Anti-inflammatory: prednisolone.

Eye-drops or guttae pro oculis (p. 216)

The drops which are applied to the eye are called guttae.

e.g. Atropine sulphate eye-drops (*Guttae atropinae sulphatis*).

Sulphacetamide eye-drops (*Guttae sulphacetamidi*).

Eye ointments or oculenta

Eye ointments are generally weaker than those applied to other surfaces and contain special drugs of value in eye conditions. They should be applied to the conjunctiva of the lower lid from special tubes or on a sterile glass rod.

e.g. Atropine eye ointment (*Oculentum atropinae*).

Mercuric oxide eye ointment (*Oculentum hydrargyri oxidi flavum*, Golden eye ointment).

Sulphacetamide eye ointment (*Oculentum sulphacetamidi*).

Gargles or gargarismata

These are fluid preparations used for gargling and are generally similar to or identical with mouth washes.

Granules

e.g. Methyl Cellulose ('Celevac'). 'Senokot'.

Inhalations (vapours) or inhalationes (vapores)

These are solutions of antiseptic or aromatic drugs or drugs themselves which are volatile or become volatile when poured into hot water.

e.g. Creosote, pine oil, menthol, and Friar's balsam (*Tinctura benzoini composita*) are often used as inhalants.

Anaesthetics such as chloroform, ether and nitrous oxide gas and drugs like amyl nitrite are also given by inhalation.

Injections or injectiones

These are sterile solutions of drugs, generally in water but sometimes in oil or other media. They are intended for subcutaneous, intramuscular and, sometimes, intravenous administration.

e.g. Mersalyl injection (*Injectio mersalyli*), intramuscular.

Morphine sulphate injection (*Injectio morphinae sulphatis*), subcutaneous.

In its wide sense the term injection includes:

1. Intradermal (into the skin).
2. Hypodermic or subcutaneous.
3. Intramuscular.
4. Intravenous.
5. Intra-peritoneal.
6. Intrathecal (into the subarachnoid space).
7. Also rectal, vaginal and urethral injections.

N.B. Almost all subcutaneous injections may also be given intramuscularly but not vice versa.

Insufflations or insufflationes

These are fine powders blown by a special insufflator directly on to the skin, the mucous membrane of the nose (e.g. Pituitary, posterior, lobe, insufflation,) or throat or a wound.

Linctuses or lincti (p. 116)

A linctus is a syrupy or viscous preparation used to allay coughing. The usual dose is 4 to 8 ml. (60 to 120 minims).

e.g. Codeine linctus (*Linctus codeinae*).
Squill opiate linctus (*Linctus scillae opiatus*).

Liniments or linimenta

The term embrocation is also used to describe the oily soapy or spirituous preparations which are applied to or rubbed into the skin and have a counter-irritant action. They must be labelled "For external use only" and are generally supplied in bottles of characteristic shape and colour so that the risk of giving them internally by mistake is reduced.

e.g. Camphor liniment (*Linimentum camphorae*, known also as Camphorated oil).
Soap liniment (*Linimentum saponis*).
Methyl salicylate liniment (*Linimentum methylis salicylatis*).

Lotions or lotiones

Lotions are watery or alcoholic solutions of drugs for external application to the skin or mucous membranes. They are generally applied on lint or similar fabric (see also Eye lotions, Mouth washes, and Nasal douches, p. 120).

e.g. Calamine lotion (*Lotio calaminae*).
Boric acid lotion (*Lotio acidi borici*).
Lead lotion (*Lotio plumbi*).

Lozenges or trochisci

These are solid flat tablets containing drugs incorporated in a gum or sugar basis. They dissolve slowly and are intended to be sucked. They usually have an astringent or antiseptic action on the mucous membrane of the mouth and throat.

e.g. Liquorice lozenges (*Trochiscis glycyrrhizae*, Brompton lozenges).
Benzocaine compound lozenges (*Trochisci benzocainae compositi*).

Mixtures or misturae

The mixture is one of the most common methods of administering medicines by mouth. Mixtures are liquid preparations of one or more drugs, generally flavoured and made up with water to a standard dose of 10 ml. or 5 ml. for children. The actual composition of standard mixtures varies somewhat in different hospitals and may be altered at will by the doctor to contain the desired dose of the component drugs. The constituents are not fully dissolved in every case and, therefore, the bottle must always be carefully shaken before administration.

e.g. Magnesium trisilicate mixture (*Mistura magnesii trisilicatis*).
Potassium citrate mixture (*Mistura potassii citratis*).
Compound senna mixture (*Mistura sennae composait*, Black draught).

Mouth Wash

Nasal Drops

Ointments or unguenta

Ointments are semi-solid preparations containing drugs mixed with materials such as soft paraffin ('Vaseline'), lard, wool fat or Lanette wax. They are intended to be spread on or rubbed into the skin.

e.g. Zinc ointment (*Unguentum zinci oxidi*).
Hydrocortisone ointment.

Paints or pigmenta

These are liquid preparations applied to the skin or mucous membranes by means of a brush. They are often antiseptic in action.

e.g. Iodine compound paint (*Pigmentum iodi compositum*, Mandl's paint).
Crystal violet paint.

Others are caustic:

e.g. Chromic acid paint (*Pigmentum acidi chromici*).

Some are used as adhesive varnishes:

e.g. Iodoform compound paint (*Pigmentum iodoformi compositum*, Whitehead's varnish*).

Pastes or pastae

These are preparations similar to ointments but often having a starchy or glycerin basis. They are generally stiffer and more solid than ointments and their ingredients are, therefore, less easily absorbed. They help to absorb secretions and are not easily rubbed off.

e.g. Starch paste (*Pasta amyli*).

Zinc and gelatin paste (*Pasta gelatini zinci*), Unna's paste.

Coal tar paste (*Pasta picis carbonis*).

Pessaries or pessi

A pessary is a cone-shaped mass containing a medicament for introduction into the vagina. It is usually made of cacao butter (oil of theobroma) or gelatin base, which remains solid at atmospheric temperature but is melted by the heat of the body.

e.g. Lactic acid pessary (*Pessus acidi lactici*).

Acetarsol pessary (*Pessus acetarsolis*).

Nasal bougies (*buginaria*) and urethral bougies (*cereoli*) are pencil-shaped structures of similar composition.

Pills or pilulae

Pills are solid spherical bodies containing medicinal agents intended to be swallowed whole and later to dissolve in the alimentary tract. They may be coated with sugar, gelatin or varnish to hide any disagreeable taste.

e.g. Aloes pill (*Pilula aloes*).

Compound rhubarb pill (*Pilula rhei composita*).

Poultices or cataplasmata

These are soft, pasty external applications used to provide heat and moisture to an inflamed or painful part.

e.g. Kaolin poultice (*Cataplasma kaolini*).

Powders or pulveres

These are mixtures of finely powdered drugs for internal use when they are usually dispensed in folded paper or capsules. A very small dose of a drug is difficult to handle in powder form and in such cases the bulk of the powder is made up of some other inert substance.

    e.g. Magnesium trisilicate compound powder.

       Pancreatin powder, strong.

Special-purpose sterile solutions

Sterile solutions are available in 1-litre bottles for two special purposes:

    1. *Intravenous infusion*

       e.g. Normal saline (Sodium Chloride Injection), 5% dextrose (Dextrose Injection).

           Dextrose–saline (Sodium Chloride and Dextrose Injection), and Dextran Injections.

    2. *Peritoneal dialysis*

       e.g. 'Dialaflex' solutions, numbers 61 (normal) and 62 (hypertonic).

Spirits or spiritus

Spirits are alcoholic solutions of oils or volatile substances which are only slightly soluble in water.

    e.g. Aromatic spirit of ammonia (*Spiritus ammonii aromaticus,* Sal volatile).

       Surgical spirit.

Spray solutions or nebulae

These are solutions of drugs intended to be sprayed on the skin or mucous membranes by means of an atomizer or aerosol.

    e.g. **For the skin:**

       Oxytetracycline-hydrocortisone ('Terra-Cortril') spray.

       For the nose:

       Ephedrine spray (*Nebula ephedrinae aquosa*).

       Xylometazoline ('Otrivine') spray.

       For the bronchi:

       Adrenaline and atropine compound spray (*Nebula adrenalinae et atropinae composita*).

       Isoprenaline spray (*Nebula isoprenalinae*).

Suppositories or suppositoria

These are conical solid bodies, not unlike pessaries, containing drugs in a basis of cacao butter (oil of theobroma) or gelatin for insertion into the rectum.

e.g. Glycerin suppository (*Suppositorium glycerini*).
Bisacodyl suppository (*Suppos. bisacodyli*), 'Dulcolax'.
Aminophylline suppository.

Syrups or syrupi

These are fluid preparations of drugs in solutions of sugar.

e.g. Syrup of orange (*Syrupus aurantii*).
Syrup of chloral (*Syrupus chloralis*).
Compound syrup of figs (*Syrupus ficorum compositus*).

Syrup of iron phosphate with quinine and strychnine (*Syrups ferri phosphatis cum quinina et strychnina*, Easton's syrup).
Compound syrup of iron phosphate (*Syrupus ferri phosphatis compositus*, Parrish's Food).

Tablets or tabellae (tablettae)

Tablets consist of drugs compressed in a mould. Many drugs intended to be dissolved in sterile water for hypodermic injection were formerly supplied in tablet form. As a general rule tablets to be taken by mouth should be crushed before administration and given with a draught of water. Some tablets, e.g. *Tabellae glycerylis trinitratis* (p. 91) are allowed to dissolve under the tongue.

e.g. Acetysalicylic acid tablets (*Tabellae acidi acetyl salicylici*, Aspirin tablets).

Vapours or vapores

These are similar to inhalations.

Vitrellae

Glass capsules to be crushed and the vapour inhaled.
e.g. Amyl nitrite vitrellae.

Confections or Confectiones

Jam-like preparations in which drugs are mixed with sugar, syrup or honey are known by this name.

e.g. Confection of senna (*Confectio sennae*).

Draughts

Extracts or Extracta

By the concentration of various vegetable or animal materials either a solid (*Extractum siccum*) or a liquid extract (*Extractum liquidum*) can be made. The liquid extracts are used in the preparation of medicines given in mixture form, while solid extracts are used for pills and tablets.

e.g. Extract of belladonna (*Extractum belladonnae*).

Extract of cascara sagrada (*Extractum cascarae sagradae*).

Glycerins or Glycerina

These are solutions of various substances in glycerin which, being sticky, has the property of adhering to mucous membranes. They may be used in the treatment of affections of the mouth and throat.

e.g. Glycerin of tannic acid (*Glycerinum acidi tannici*).

Glycerin of borax (*Glycerinum boracis*).

Glycerin of phenol (*Glycerinum phenolis*).

Medicated waters or Aquae

These usually contain some volatile substance or oil in solution. A number of them are used as flavouring agents.

e.g. Chloroform water (*Aqua chloroformi*).

Peppermint water (*Aqua menthae piperitae*).

Musilages or Mucilagines

These are viscous aqueous solutions of gums used for the suspension of insoluble drugs.

e.g. Mucilage of acacia (*Mucilago acaciae*).

Mucilage of tragacanth (*Mucilago tragacanthae*).

Oils or Olea

With the exception of liquid paraffin, which is a mineral oil, and the fish-liver oils, the oils are obtained by distillation or expression from vegetable substances.

e.g. Almond oil (*Oleum amygdalae*).

Peanut oil (*Oleum arachis*).

Oil of clove (*Oleum caryophylli*).

Linseed oil (*Oleum lini*).

Olive oil (*Oleum olivae*).

Castor oil (*Oleum ricini*).

Pastilles or pastilli

These are sweet-like preparations which should be dissolved slowly in the mouth.

Plasters or emplastra

Plasters consist of medical substances mixed with lead soap, oil, rubber or resin, and spread on coarse muslin or similar material. They adhere to the skin at body temperature and are usually warmed slightly before application. They are mostly employed as counter-irritants, but may produce blistering on sensitive skins.

Solution-tablets or solvellae

These are compressed tablets intended to be dissolved in water to make up solutions. Tablets of a given dosage dissolved in an appropriate amount of water make up solutions of standard strength.

    e.g. Mercury iodide solution-tablets (*Solvellae hydrargyri iodidi*, Biniodide tablets).

        Mercury perchloride solution-tablets (*Solvellae hydrargyri perchloridi*).

Tinctures or tincturae

These are solutions of crude drugs in alcohol and resemble spirits but differ from them in their mode of preparation. Their individual doses differ considerably.

    e.g. Tincture of belladonna (*Tinctura belladonnae*).

        Compound tincture of benzoin (*Tinctura benzoini composita*, Friar's balsam).

        Tincture of digitalis (*Tinctura digitalis*).

CHAPTER 3

The Administration of Drugs

Therapeutic substances are administered or applied in a number of different ways.

1. **Via the alimentary tract**
   (a) By the mouth (*per os*)

Capsules	Mixtures containing:
Draughts	Extracts
Elixirs	Mucilages
Linctuses	Oils
Lozenges	Solid drugs
Pastilles	Solutions (liquores)
Pills	Spirits
Powders	Tinctures
Tablets	Waters (aquae)

   (b) Sublingual tablets (under the tongue).
   (c) By the rectum (*per rectum*)

   Enemas   Suppositories

2. **Via the respiratory tract**
   Inhalations including anaethetics
   Sprays   Aerosols   Vapours

3. **Via the uro-genital tract**
   (a) By the urethra (*per urethram*)
   Bougies   Injections
   (b) By the vagina (*per vaginam*)
   Douches   Pessaries

4. **Drugs applied to the skin**
   (a) Local applications:

Collodions	Liniments	Pastes
Creams	Lotions	Plasters

    Dusting powders   Ointments
    Glycerins   Paints

(*b*) Baths.

(*c*) Ionization.

5. Drugs applied to mucous membranes

Many of the above may also be applied to mucous membranes. In addition:

  (*a*) Mucous membrane of the mouth:

      Gargles   Mouth washes (collutoria)
      Lozenges   Pastilles

  (*b*) Mucous membrane of the nose:

      Inhalations   Nasal douches (collunaria)
      Insufflations   Sprays

  (*c*) The eye:

      Eye discs (lamellae)   Eye ointments (oculenta)
      Eye drops (guttae)   Eye washes (collyria)

  (*d*) The ear:

      Ear drops (auristillae)   Insufflations

6. Drugs given by injection

  (*a*) Intradermal (into the skin).

      e.g. BCG vaccine

      Tuberculin tests, e.g. Mantoux

  (*b*) Hypodermic or subcutaneous. (Into the loose tissue spaces just beneath the skin.)

      e.g. Narcotic drugs such as morphine

      Insulin

  (*b*) Intramuscular or into a muscle, e.g. paraldehyde.

  (*d*) Intravenous or into a vein, e.g. hydrocortisone.

  (*e*) Intrathecal or into the spinal canal.

      e.g. Penicillin, streptomycin. (N.B. Small doses).

      Spinal anaesthetics

The term "parenteral" means "not through the alimentary canal" and is used to imply some type of injection.

Injections are customarily given with a syringe and needle, both of which may be disposable. However, mass inoculation programmes can be more rapidly completed with a pressure injector, e.g. the Porton Jet Injector. This delivers drugs in a high-velocity jet which painlessly penetrates unbroken skin and deposits the drugs intradermally, subcutaneously or intramuscularly.

Up to 800 inoculations per hour are possible with this instrument.

TECHNIQUE OF ADMINISTRATION

Rules for the oral administration of drugs

The administration of drugs is a matter of great importance to the nurse and is one of the routine duties which carries with it great responsibility.

Many drugs are powerful poisons; while doses of others are carefully calculated in order to produce the desired effect.

Absolute accuracy of measurement in every case is essential and is an important part of a nurse's training. Familiarity should never lead to carelessness. In the event of any doubt entering the nurse's mind about the correctness of a dose of the drug she is about to give, there must be no hesitation in referring the matter to a senior officer.

Points to remember about administering medicines are:

1. Punctuality, with special regard to the instructions before and after meals and special directions, e.g. "with water".
(Medicines so ordered should be given 20 minutes before meals or immediately after meals.)

2. Read the label on the bottle and check the drug and dose with the patient's treatment card.

3. Make a habit of shaking the bottle in each case, irrespective of whether the medicine is clear or containing a sediment. This should be done by inverting the bottle several times, with the forefinger on the cork to prevent accidental spilling.

4. Measure the dose carefully into a suitable medicine measure. Modern mixtures are made up to doses of 10 ml. (5 ml. for children). The measure should, if possible, be read while it is standing on a flat surface. If not, it must be held at eye level, taking care not to tilt the measure either backwards or forwards, a movement which will obviously produce an inaccurate reading.

It is not a wise practice to rely on the marking often found on medicine bottles and is certainly bad training.

5. Hold the cork with the little finger while pouring out.

6. Give the medicine or tablet to the patient immediately and watch him take it.

It is the proud boast of some patients that they pour all their medicine down the sink. Do not leave drugs lying about or permit unauthorized persons to handle them. In a private house circumstances may, of course, modify this procedure.

7. Observe and report any signs of overdose, reaction or intolerance. In this connection, if any mistake should unfortunately be made in the administration of a drug either by giving the wrong drug or dose, the nurse must immediately report the fact, irrespective of any possible consequences to herself. An error reported at once can sometimes be rectified without serious consequences to the patient.

8. Have all hypodermic injections and dangerous drugs checked by a second person and enter the dose given in the poison register when this is required.

9. Try to make the administration of unpleasant drugs as agreeable as possible, e.g. give iron mixtures with a straw to prevent blackening of the teeth, and give the patient an opportunity of brushing the teeth without delay. Sweets, fruit juice, a mouth-wash or a piece of bread may help to remove a disagreeable taste.

10. Keep medicine bottles clean by wiping after use and always pour out of the side away from the label, i.e. keep the label uppermost.

11. Remember that tablets and capsules are supplied in various strengths and, therefore the labelled dose must be carefully checked with the treatment card.

Notes on the administration of drugs

Linctus: Should be sipped slowly.

Lozenge and *pastille:* Should be sucked slowly.

Mixture: See that the patient takes any sediment which tends to collect in the medicine glass.

Pill, capsule: Should be given with a drink of water and swallowed whole.

Cachet: Should be soaked in water before swallowing.

Oil: Occasionally two or three drops of a volatile oil, such as oil of peppermint, are ordered for flatulence and are best given on a cube of sugar.

Olive oil, arachis oil and liquid paraffin are given by mouth in the usual way, preferably using a porcelain measure.

Suppository: This should be inserted into the rectum with the patient in the lateral position. It may be dipped in warm water (the purpose being to melt the surface of the suppository) to facilitate introduction, which should be carried out slowly with the gloved finger, taking care to pass the suppository through the anal sphincter into the rectum.

Bougie: Dip in warm oil or water before insertion.

Pessary: Slight moistening may be necessary before insertion into the vagina, but usually there is sufficient mucous secretion present to make introduction easy.

Powder: (i) The contents of a paper may be placed on the back of the patient's tongue and followed by a drink of milk or water.

(ii) Sprinkle on the surface of a little milk.

(iii) Mix with jam in a sandwich for children.

(iv) Effervescent powders should be stirred in half a tumbler of water and taken at once, e.g. Seidlitz powder.

Tablet: As a rule a tablet should be swallowed whole but some may be crushed, placed on the back of the tongue and swallowed with a draught of water.

Tablets of glyceryl trinitrate and isoprenaline should be allowed to dissolve under the tongue, i.e. sublingually.

Antacid tablets (e.g. 'Gelusil') should be allowed to dissolve slowly in the mouth.

THE ACTION OF DRUGS

It will be clear from consideration of the enormous number of drugs at our disposal and the divers conditions for which they may be employed, that no very precise summary can be given of their mode of action. However, among the ways in which drugs can act are:

1. The direct action on micro-organisms and parasites on the surface of the body or on other objects.

    e.g. The use of antiseptics for sterilizing instruments or as lotions applied externally; benzyl benzoate emulsion applied for scabies.

2. By giving drugs which have a direct lethal effect on organisms within the tissues of the body.

    e.g. (*a*) The use of chemotherapy (sulphonamides, etc.) and antibiotics, such as penicillin, against bacteria which are sensitive to their action.

        (*b*) Chloroquine and similar drugs for malaria.

3. By producing some direct and obvious chemical effect.

    e.g. (*a*) Neutralizing the hydrochloric acid in the gastric juice by giving antacids such as magnesium trisilicate or aluminium hydroxide.

        (*b*) Turning an acid urine alkaline by giving potassium citrate; or an alkaline urine acid with acid sodium phosphate.

4. Producing the desired effect by some definite physiological action which can be clearly explained by a knowledge of the actual processes which normally occur.

    e.g. Atropine paralyses the nerve endings to the muscle of the pupil of the eye and its administration results in dilatation of the pupil. On the other hand, physostigmine ('Eserine') stimulates the nerve endings and its action is opposite to that of atropine, for it causes the pupil to contract.

B

The action of digitalis on the conducting tissues of the heart in the bundle of His, whereby it blocks a number of the frequent and irregular impulses coming from the atrium (auricle) in atrial fibrillation, is also a good example.

5. Drugs may be given to replace some missing factor which should normally be supplied by the body. Such drugs are usually chemically identical with the missing substance and are either made in the laboratory or obtained from some suitable animal.

e.g. (*a*) Insulin to supply the missing pancreatic hormone in diabetes. Various ductless gland preparations e.g. thyroid, pituitary and ovarian extracts.

(*b*) Vitamin B_{12} by injection to replace that which cannot be absorbed from the diet in pernicious anaemia.

6. Vitamins, and drugs like iron and calcium given to supply dietetic deficiencies. Iron and calcium may also be required when their absorption is defective.

7. Many other examples might be given, but they will become apparent as individual drugs are considered.

A **placebo** is a medicine given to please or satisfy a patient without having any special pharmacological effect. It is really, therefore, a form of psychotherapy.

Idiosyncrasy

Idiosyncrasy may be defined as an abnormal or unusual response to a normal dose of a drug. (The word is derived from the Greek: *idios*=one's own, *syncrasis*=blending.) It is a form of over-sensitivity which is sometimes due to allergy: in fact, the term "drug allergy" is sometimes used.

It is only met with in isolated cases, but, in such instances, an ordinary dose may produce toxic symptoms which are unpleasant, alarming or even dangerous. The symptoms manifested may be similar to those seen when an overdose of the drug has been taken by a normal person.

The symptoms may appear immediately, particularly after injections, but may be delayed for some hours or even days.

Since the nurse may administer the drug herself or the patient will be under her observation after it has been given, the subject is clearly one of great importance to her. Any unusual symptoms occurring after a drug has been taken should, therefore, be reported without delay. The condition may develop after a drug has been given internally, but not infrequently external applications to the skin produce severe local reactions. Sometimes a patient is aware of the sensitivity and gives information on the subject beforehand.

The most common types of reaction which occur are:

1. Rashes and skin eruptions.

2. General symptoms including collapse, nausea, vomiting and giddiness.

3. Aplastic anaemia and agranulocytosis, due to an unexpected toxic action of the drug in the bone marrow. These are serious conditions which may prove fatal (see p. 103).

While it is difficult to exclude any particular drugs, the following are important:

1. *Quinine*, causing deafness, giddiness, headache, nausea, shivering, noises in the head, disturbances of vision and transient rashes such as urticaria or erythema.

2. *Sodium salicylate and aspirin*, causing noises in the head (tinnitus), deafness, malaise, nausea, rapid pulse or an erythematous rash.

N.B.—Aspirin occasionally causes haematemesis or melaena, and may also produce serious reactions in asthmatics.

3. *Potassium iodide*, causes increased secretion from the respiratory tract resembling a severe cold in the head, laryngitis and skin eruptions similar to acne. Iodine given internally in other forms may produce the same effects (iodism).

4. *Bromides*. Skin eruptions such as pustular acne or erythema are the most common manifestations. Mental dullness and general weakness may also be present. The symptoms of bromism resemble iodism and there may be an increase in the mucous secretion from the respiratory tract.

5. *Calomel*. This may produce symptoms of severe collapse in some individuals but is rarely used.

6. *Cocaine* (including procaine, 'Novocain', etc.). Malaise, vomiting, pyrexia; collapse with pallor, rapid pulse and slow respirations, and sometimes convulsions or fits, may all occur. Death occasionally follows from respiratory paralysis.

7. *Sulphonamides*. Drugs of this group may produce serious symptoms in some individuals, e.g. changes in the white cells of the blood (agranulocytosis), haematuria, pyrexia after the initial lesion for which the drug has been given has subsided (drug fever), and skin rashes (see p. 229).

8. *Penicillin* and *Ampicillin* sometimes cause rashes or even

severe collapse in sensitive persons, and streptomycin may also
give rise to troublesome eruptions in those who handle it.

Tolerance

This may be of two types: (i) *Natural* tolerance, which is really
the direct opposite of idiosyncrasy and implies that the individual
resists the action of a certain drug and can tolerate much larger
doses than a normal person; (ii) *Acquired*. This means a state
induced in the normal person by the prolonged use of a drug
whereby he can gradually tolerate increasing doses which would,
if administered in the first place, have produced toxic symptoms.

Tolerance is a common phenomenon and is exhibited by a
number of drugs. Tobacco and alcohol are obvious examples. The
first cigarette may produce nausea, vomiting and a greenish pallor
of the skin, while a seasoned smoker may consume up to fifty
cigarettes a day without any immediately obvious symptoms,
except perhaps a well-deserved "smoker's cough". The difference
in effect between two persons consuming the same amount of
alcohol is also well known.

Among the important drugs used in therapeutics for which
tolerance may be acquired are: opium and morphine, atropine
and belladonna, stramonium and arsenic (p. 146).

It must always be remembered however, that when a drug is
discontinued the acquired tolerance is usually lost and, if the drug
is re-commenced at a later date, ordinary doses must be used.

It is not known what acquired tolerance depends on. It may be
that some chemical "antibody" is formed or that the tissues fail
to absorb the drug fully. In some cases the excretion may be more
rapid, in others the drug is more quickly destroyed or converted
into some inert substance.

Drug addiction

The World Health Organisation prefers the more comprehensive
term *"drug dependence"* to "addiction" and "habit". Dependence
may be *emotional* (psychic) or *physical* or both. If there is physical
dependence the patient becomes physically ill on withdrawal of
the drug (withdrawal syndrome) since some of the metabolic
processes of the body come to depend on the drug. The *types of
drug dependence* (W.H.O.) are as follows:

    Morphine-type (includes heroin and opium)
    Barbiturate- or alcohol-type

Amphetamine-type
Cocaine-type
Hallucinogen-type (e.g. LSD)
Cannabis-type (marijuana) (p. 150)

In all of these there is a degree of emotional dependence but only in the first two types is there physical dependence. Patients are sometimes dependent on a mixture of drugs, e.g. barbiturate–amphetamine or heroin–cocaine mixtures. Any substances on the D.D.A. list may induce dependence, and so may many drugs which act on the central nervous system and which are classified as Fourth Schedule Poisons.

Treatment is notoriously difficult and involves the gradual withdrawal of the drug. In the case of heroin dependence, methadone may be substituted; methadone dependence is less objectionable. When cure of drug dependency is impossible the drugs may be supplied under supervision. Only doctors working in special treatment centres may prescribe heroin or cocaine for addiction; for the treatment of organic disease any doctor may, of course, prescribe these drugs.

This is a state in which the individual acquires a craving for a particular drug, often to such an extent that life becomes unbearable without it.

Cumulative effect

When a drug is taken one of two things may happen.

(a) It may be destroyed or converted into some inert or inactive substance by the tissues, especially the liver.

(b) It may be excreted unchanged by the kidneys, bowel, lungs or skin.

Clearly there will be a definite relationship for each drug, between the rate at which it is taken in and the rate of its destruction or excretion and, as a rule, the dosage and intervals at which any drug is administered are adjusted to meet this situation. It follows that if the rate of administration is greater than the rate of destruction or excretion, the drug will accumulate in the tissues and increase in amount with each dose taken.

Some drugs are especially liable to show this phenomenon and will produce the symptoms of overdosage or poisoning.

Digitalis is an important example. Mercury, arsenic and lead are others. In lead poisoning, small quantities of lead may be absorbed into the body over a long period and, finally, when a certain concentration exists in the tissues the typical symptoms appear, e.g. colic and various types of paralysis.

Drug interaction

Sometimes one drug will increase the effects of another if taken at the same time (potentiation) and the results may be dangerous.

e.g. (i) Alcohol increases the effect of barbiturates, an important factor when driving a car.

(ii) The action of digitalis is enhanced by thiazide diuretics which increase potassium excretion.

(iii) Dangerous results occur if a patient taking a monoamine oxidase inhibitor (MAOI), e.g. phenelzine ('Nardil', etc., see p 152), has cheese in his diet.

(iv) Aspirin and phenylbutazone increase the activity of anticoagulant drugs.

(v) Sulphonamides should be avoided in diabetics taking tolbutamide, which is a sulphonamide derivative.

DOSAGE OF DRUGS IN CHILDHOOD

Drugs are prescribed for children on the basis of their weight or body surface area (B.S.A.). Sometimes one basis is preferable, sometimes the other. For example, atropine is best prescribed for an infant by reference to weight since dosage based on surface area may be excessive. Except for under-weight children, drugs are often prescribed on an age basis. No method of prescribing drugs for children is perfect and a nurse should always be on the look-out for possible adverse effects.

Many medicines are available in liquid form (suspensions or elixirs). It cannot be too strongly emphasized that liquids should be thoroughly shaken before a dose is measured out from the bottle. All B.N.F. liquid medicines (linctuses, elixirs and paediatric mixtures) should be made up by the dispenser for individual patients so that the correct dose is contained in a 5 ml. teaspoonful.

The nurse may encounter various formulae used in the calculation of dosage of drugs for children. They include *Young's formula* in which the dose for children less than 12 years of age may be obtained by dividing the age by age+12. Thus for a child of 6:

$$6 \div (6+12) = \tfrac{1}{3}$$

therefore one-third of the usual adult dose would be given.

Catzel's formula

$$\frac{\text{B.S.A. of child}}{\text{B.S.A. of adult}} \times 100 = \% \text{ of adult dose.}$$

TABLE 1.

Age	Weight (kg.)	(lb.)	% age of adult dose
Birth	3·2	7	12·5
2 months	4·5	10	15
4 ,,	6·5	14	20
12 ,,	10	22	25
18 ,,	11	24	30
5 years	18	40	40
7 ,,	23	50	50
10 ,,	30	66	60
11 ,,	36	80	70
12 ,,	40	88	75
14 ,,	45	100	80
16 ,,	54	120	90
Adult	65	145	100

Some drugs are prescribed for adults on the basis of mg per kg of body weight. The appropriate dose for a child may be calculated by taking age into account.

For a child under 1 year, the dose calculated on a weight basis should be multiplied by 2. It should be multiplied by 1·5 for a child between 1 and 7 years and by 1·25 for a child of 12 years.

Weight and body surface area are not the only factors on which suitable dosage depends. Children tolerate the following drugs well and larger doses can be given than would be suggested by application of the formulae:

Aperients   Hyoscyamus   Sulphonamides

On the other hand, some drugs are badly tolerated and smaller doses are necessary. Morphine, opium and other narcotics fall into this category.

In old age, too, it is usually advisable to reduce the average dose somewhat. Doses of digitalis preparations which would be therapeutic in younger adults may be seriously toxic in elderly people. A special low-dosage form of digoxin, containing only 0·625 mg in each tablet, has therefore been marketed under the name of 'Lanoxin PG', PG meaning paediatric–geriatric.

CHAPTER 4

Disinfectants and Antiseptics

Only a section of the large subject of sterilization falls within the province of Materia Medica, namely, the killing of bacteria, viruses, fungi, etc. by chemical methods. This presents three problems:

1. The killing of organisms away from the human body, viz. the sterilization of instruments, utensils, linen, dressings, excreta, etc.

2. The killing of organisms on the surface of the body and in wounds.

3. The killing of organisms within the tissues of the body by drugs given by internal administration. (See Chapter 18.)

Methods of sterilization

The following methods of killing or removing organisms may be employed:

I. Physical methods

(a) *Heat*. (i) Ordinary boiling for periods up to 20 minutes depending on the nature of the article. Two minutes boiling kills most bacteria, but spores are not necessarily destroyed by the most prolonged boiling.

The addition of 2% washing soda to the water is more lethal to the bacteria and spores.

(ii) Steam under pressure, as produced in the autoclave.

(iii) Dry heat which is not so effective as moist heat and, in comparison, requires to be of a higher temperature and to act for longer periods.

(b) *Radiation*. Direct exposure to sunlight or ultra-violet rays is effective in destroying a number of organisms. Gamma-irradiation is now frequently used for sterilizing surgical materials (e.g. sutures).

(c) *Filtration.* It is possible to remove bacteria from water and other fluids by passing them through a special very fine filter of the Berkefeld and Pasteur–Chamberland type. Viruses are smaller than ordinary bacteria and will pass through such filters, hence the term "filter-passing virus" is sometimes used.

II. Chemical methods

The majority of these drugs owe their germicidal or antiseptic action to one of the following properties:

1. The power to extract water from the bodies of bacteria.
2. The power of coagulating proteins.
3. A general poisonous action on protein.
4. The liberation of oxygen.

The value of soap and detergents as aids to disinfection should not be overlooked. Most of them have no germicidal power in themselves but, when used on the hands or other articles, very efficiently remove the superficial layer of grease in which bacteria are lodged, and so facilitate the subsequent application of germicides. Very few disinfectant substances can be combined with toilet soap and the majority of the "carbolic soaps" are useless from a germicidal point of view. On the other hand, Lysol, a solution of cresol in soap, is a powerful germicide. The detergent cetrimide ('Cetavlon') has mild antiseptic properties. For washing the hands before performing surgical procedures, hexachlorophane ('Phisohex') or povidone–iodine ('Betadine') may be used instead of plain soap. The patients' skin may be swabbed with cetrimide, surgical spirit, tincture of iodine or povidone–iodine prior to operation.

Whenever possible, sterilization of instruments and utensils by boiling is to be preferred to chemical methods, while the autoclave is indispensable for dressings and gloves.

The main uses for chemical disinfectants in this connection are to keep sterile instruments free from further contamination; in emergency when other methods are not available and for non-boilable appliances, e.g. gum-elastic catheters and some electrical connections.

The disinfection of lavatories and drains is practically impossible and most disinfectant fluids poured down them only act as cleansing agents and deodorants.

DISINFECTANTS AND ANTISEPTICS

Strictly speaking, an antiseptic is a substance which prevents the growth of micro-organisms but does not necessarily kill them, so that their growth may be possible after the removal of the drug. Such action is sometimes described as **bacteriostatic**. A disinfectant or germicide kills bacteria and, by comparison with antiseptics, may be called **bactericidal**. All disinfectants are, therefore, antiseptics, but an antiseptic is not necessarily a germicide.

The term antiseptic is generally used for agents applied to living surfaces, while disinfectants are those used on inanimate objects.

It must be remembered, however, that a substance in strong concentration may be germicidal, but in weaker solutions may only act as an antiseptic, so that no exact distinction can be made between the two terms.

The following is a summary of some of the important factors upon which disinfectant and antiseptic action depends:

1. The strength of the disinfectant.
2. The time for which it acts.
3. The temperature.
4. The nature of the material in which it has to act. The presence of pus or other organic matter retards the action of some drugs of this class.
5. The type of the infecting organisms.

1. The strength of the disinfectant. It has just been mentioned that a substance in strong concentration may be bactericidal but in weaker solutions may only act as an antiseptic, i.e. as a bacteriostatic.

This is a most important fact to realize, for many of the drugs of this group are used in various strengths for different purposes, and dilution affects each disinfectant to a markedly different degree.

Thus, phenol in concentrated form acts very rapidly, in dilutions up to 1 in 100 it acts with reasonable rapidity but in solutions weaker than this is almost ineffective and organisms will survive for many hours in a strength of 1 in 150. In other words the phenol in a "Carbolic bath", formerly given at the end of an infectious illness, was quite useless.

2. The time of action. Speaking generally, this varies with the concentration of the drug. The stronger the solution of the drug, the shorter the time required to kill bacteria.

The dyes, mercury salts and the salts of other metals tend to be slow in action, whereas disinfectants dependent upon the liberation of chlorine are relatively rapid.

3. Temperature. The action of disinfectants is, in most instances, increased to some extent by a rise in temperature. Therefore, preparations for external use should be employed at body temperature whenever possible.

4. The nature of the material. This specially applies to the presence of pus, blood and other organic matter, such as necrotic tissue, which tend to decrease the activity of many antiseptics and germicides.

5. The type of the infecting organism. The most powerful disinfectants are germicidal to all organisms. On the other hand, some disinfectants, as well as the more powerful ones in weaker concentrations, show what may be called "selective action". That is, a disinfectant may be more effective against one organism than another.

For example, staphylococci are very susceptible to crystal (gentian) violet dye. Dyes of the flavine group are more active against streptococci than staphylococci. These facts may be of importance in the dressing and irrigation of wounds.

IMPORTANT DISINFECTANTS AND ANTISEPTICS

Much research has been carried out on these agents. The great difficulty has been to produce those which can be used not only outside the body but also on the human tissues, because so many substances which are lethal to bacteria also injure the tissues and are, therefore, of no value in disinfecting the skin or irrigating wounds, for they will do more harm than good.

The ideal requirements for a disinfectant are:

1. To be strongly lethal to bacteria but non-injurious to human tissues (i.e. non-toxic and non-corrosive).

2. To be easily soluble in water, saline and serum, and to act efficiently in the presence of pus, blood or dead tissue.

3. To be inexpensive.

The disinfectants and antiseptics most commonly used can be classified roughly into several main groups:

1. Acids and alkalis.
2. Solutions of certain metallic salts.
3. Various organic compounds (including alcohols and coal-tar products, etc.).

4. The halogens.
5. Oxidizing agents.
6. Dyes.   (*a*) Aniline type;   (*b*) Flavine type.
7. Various other substances, ethylene oxide gas sterilization, etc.

1. ACIDS AND ALKALIS

Strong mineral acids (such as nitric, sulphuric and hydrochloric acids) and alkalis (caustic potash and caustic soda) are corrosive and destroy all living matter. They also dissolve or damage many substances in common use. They are, therefore, unsuitable for application as disinfectants either to the surface of the body or on utensils in concentrated form.

They have been occasionally employed as caustics (i.e. to burn away tissue), for example, the application of strong nitric acid to warts.

In appropriate dilution they are sometimes employed in treatment. It will be recalled that the gastric juice contains hydrochloric acid (1·2 per cent) and that this is sometimes referred to as the "antiseptic barrier" of the stomach. Dilute hydrochloric acid, 10 per cent [*Acidum hydrochloricum dilutum*, B.P., dose up to 4 ml. (60 minims)] is occasionally given in dyspeptic conditions and in some cases of pernicious anaemia, a disease in which hydrochloric acid is absent from the gastric juice, but is of doubtful value.

There are a number of other weak acids not belonging to the mineral acid group which are non-corrosive and used in therapeutics for other purposes. The majority are given internally and are considered later. Others are employed externally for various purposes. The following are some which are given internally:

Acetysalicylic acid (aspirin).	Lactic acid.
Ascorbic acid (Vitamin C).	Mandelic acid.
Citric acid.	Nicotinic acid.

Lactic acid is also used as an antiseptic in vaginal douches and pessaries.

Tannic acid was once used as an external application on account of its astringent properties and its power of tanning or coagulating proteins on an open surface, e.g. for burns. It has a serious toxic effect on the liver after absorption.

Boric Acid (*Acidum boricum*)

Boric acid, a white crystalline substance, is an antiseptic of feeble action which is non-irritant. A 4% lotion may be used for irrigating the eye.

Ointments and dusting powders containing more than 5% boric acid should not be applied to raw or weeping surfaces. Absorption of boric acid thus applied can have dangerous and even fatal toxic results.

It was formerly used as a preservative for food, but this is now illegal.

Salicylic acid (*Acidum salicylicum*)

This occurs as colourless crystals and has some antiseptic properties, especially against fungi. For this purpose it is used in ointments in certain

skin diseases, e.g. *Unguentum acidi salicylici compositum* (Whitfield's ointment). It is also used in foot-powders. In plasters (*Emplastrum salicylicum*)
or collodion, it is used for corns and warts.

Salicylic acid is not given internally, but its derivatives, sodium salicylate
and acetysalicylic acid (aspirin) are well known (see p. 143).

Acetic acid (*Acidum aceticum*)

This is an organic acid which is present in vinegar. Its only possible use as
an antiseptic lies in the fact that a 2 per cent solution is an effective dressing
for infections due to *Bacillus pyocyaneus* (a good example of selective action
previously mentioned).

2. SOLUTIONS OF CERTAIN METALLIC SALTS

The metallic salts which can act as disinfectants are those which
have the power of coagulating proteins, such as silver nitrate,
copper sulphate, zinc sulphate, biniodide and perchloride of
mercury.

Silver nitrate (*Argenti nitras*)

This substance has special uses and may be employed in solid
form or as a solution.

(*a*) In solid form it is used as a caustic (lunar caustic) to destroy
excess of granulation tissue in an open wound or ulcer. The stick
is slightly moistened and rubbed lightly on the area of granulation
tissue, care being taken to avoid contaminating the surrounding
skin. This process may be painful and produces a white appearance,
which later turns black. When thus applied it destroys all the
tissues and organisms with which it comes in contact.

N.B.—Silver nitrate stains on the skin may be removed by mercuric
chloride solution.

(*b*) As a solution for irrigating the bladder in chronic cystitis
the strength may be gradually increased from 1 in 10,000 to
1 in 2000.

(*c*) For eye drops and as a prophylactic against ophthalmia neonatorum in
a newborn infant, a less irritating colloidal silver preparation such as *Guttae
argentoproteini* ('Argyrol' 10 per cent), in which silver is combined with a
protein, has been used.

Copper sulphate (*Cupri sulphas*)

Copper sulphate was used in the now obsolete Benedict's test for glycosuria.

Zinc sulphate (*Zinci sulphas*)

This substance, and also zinc chloride, has been used in the form of antiseptic eye drops. It has been given by mouth (220 mg doses) in the treatment of leg ulcers.

Mercury biniodide (*Hydrargyri iodum rubrum* or Red mercuric oxide)
    This is a very poisonous antiseptic which is used externally. It may be employed in aqueous or spirituous solutions, viz.:
Aqueous solution: 1 in 2000 to 1 in 5000 for application to wounds.
                      1 in 5000 to 1 in 10,000 as a vaginal douche.
Spirituous solution: 1 in 500 to 1 in 2000 to render the skin aseptic.
    It is wise to wash out wounds or the vagina after its use with sterile water in order to prevent the risk of poisoning from the absorption of mercury.

Mercury perchloride (*Hydrargyri perchloridum*, Mercuric chloride, Corrosive
    sublimate)
    This is a colourless, poisonous, antiseptic which must not be confused with mercurous chloride (calomel). Solutions of it and mercury biniodide may be artificially coloured to minimize the risk of being mistaken for water or other harmless liquid. Its solution is used in strengths up to 1 in 1000 for external purposes, but it should not be applied to steel instruments on account of its action on the metal.
    Both mercury biniodide and perchloride are undoubtedly bacteriostatic, but their bactericidal powers are uncertain. They tend to be slow in their action, which is further retarded by the presence of blood.
    There are a number of organic mercurial antiseptics which are less toxic and less irritating than the inorganic compounds. They include mercuro-chrome and merthiolate. 'Metaphen' is a mercurial disinfectant.
    N.B.—Some skins are sensitive to mercury and its use may result in dermatitis.

3. VARIOUS ORGANIC COMPOUNDS

The alcohols
    Chemically there are a number of different alcohols but only two require special mention, viz.:
        Ethyl alcohol.
        Methyl alcohol.
Ethyl alcohol. In its pure form and when free from any trace of water it is referred to as absolute alcohol.
    Ethyl alcohol has maximum antiseptic properties as a 70 per cent solution, but in stronger or weaker concentrations is less effective. It is useful for rendering the unbroken skin aseptic, but it is painful when applied to raw surfaces and this, together with the fact that the presence of proteins reduce its activity, renders it unsuitable for application to wounds. Applied externally, however, alcohol hardens the skin and is useful in preventing bedsores. It evaporates quickly and is used in cooling lotions in the treatment of sprains

and contusions. It is the type of alcohol present in fermented beverages (p. 225) and is also the basis of a number of pharmaceutical preparations, e.g. tinctures and some liniments.

Absolute alcohol is a purer form which can only be purchased from a chemist on a prescription.

Surgical spirit is industrial methylated spirit with castor oil and other additives. Its methyl alcohol content makes it too toxic for internal use.

Methyl alcohol (Wood alcohol, Methanol). When a chronic alcoholic falls upon hard times he may take to drinking methylated spirit which is ethyl alcohol adulterated ("denatured") with methyl alcohol. Methanol is oxidized in the body to formaldehyde and then to formic acid, two very toxic substances. The symptoms of poisoning include headache, vertigo, vomiting, severe abdominal pain, back pain, muscle cramps, dyspnoea, restlessness, delirium, coma and circulatory collapse. Partial or total blindness, caused by the formaldehyde, is common and is often permanent.

In the treatment of acute methanol poisoning the most urgent measure is to combat the severe acidosis caused by the formic acid. Large quantities of sodium bicarbonate may have to be given by intravenous infusion and continued for a while orally. Ethyl alcohol may also be useful in treatment because it reduces the conversion of the methanol into toxic metabolites; the dose is 1–1·5 ml. per kg initially, followed by 0·5–1 ml. per kg two hourly for four days. Haemodialysis, if available, is a very effective treatment for acute methanol poisoning and is indicated if the above measures are unsuccessful or if the blood methanol level exceeds 50 mg per 100 ml.

The coal-tar disinfectants

A large number of chemical substances are produced from coal tar. Many have germicidal properties and a number of others have various medicinal uses. Among the most important of the former are phenol (carbolic acid) and the cresols, which are the basis of the disinfectants of the lysol type.

Phenol (*Acidium carbolicum*)

Pure phenol is a caustic which occurs in colourless crystals and has a characteristic pungent odour, but it is rarely used in this state.

Phenol is most commonly supplied in the form of a lotion (1 in 20), which may be further diluted for special purposes. It should not be employed as a dressing for open wounds as its absorption may either damage the tissues locally or cause general toxic symptoms.

A 1 in 20 solution is used for disinfecting excreta in typhoid fever and similar conditions.

Liquefied phenol (*Acidum carbolicum liquidum*) contains 80 per cent phenol and is sometimes used as a caustic. It must not be confused with *Lotio phenolis* (referred to above, which is usually of 1 in 20 strength).

Phenol is sometimes dissolved in glycerin instead of water. Solutions in glycerin are much less caustic (and of lower germicidal power) than those in water. Thus glycerin and phenol ear drops (*Auristillae phenolis*) contain 7·5 per cent of phenol but under no circumstances should these be diluted with water which will render them caustic in action. It follows that the ear must be carefully dried after syringing with lotions before glycerin and phenol drops are instilled.

Phenol also has some local anaesthetic action, hence its value as a mouth wash or gargle (*Gargarisma phenolis*) in painful affections of the mouth and throat, for which it is also employed as a lozenge. As ear drops it is, therefore, of value both on account of its antiseptic and anaesthetic properties.

Other preparations include:

Glycerin of phenol (*Glycerinum phenolis*, 16 per cent).

Phenol ointment (*Unguentum phenolis*, 3 per cent).

It should be noted that the correct modern term for this drug is PHENOL and that carbolic acid, no longer the "official" name, should be dropped.

Lysol (*Liquor cresolis saponatus*, B.P.—Solution of cresol with soap)

Lysol is a solution of cresol in soap. It is a powerful disinfectant and caustic. It may be employed undiluted for sterilizing instruments, which should be immersed for 5 minutes. Care should always be taken to avoid splashing the skin and especially the eyes, and it should be applied to utensils with a mop or by using rubber gloves. Utensils should then be rinsed with sterile water before use. Splashes of phenol or lysol on the skin should be immediately removed by swabbing with glycerin or olive oil. Water must be avoided.

Weaker solutions are also germicidal, but must be allowed to operate for longer periods.

It should not be employed on the skin in concentrations exceeding 2 per cent. For douches, a 1 per cent solution is generally employed (5 ml. in 500 ml.).

'Sudol' is a non-caustic proprietory form of lysol.

There are many proprietary preparations similar to lysol which are used for the same purposes, but in strengths appropriate for each, e.g. 'Izal' and 'Jeyes' Fluid'.

Chloroxylenol solution (*Liquor chloroxylenolis* 'Dettol', 'Roxenol') may be used (*a*) for cuts, 1 in 80, or 5 ml. in 400 ml. of water, (*b*) vaginal douche, 1 in 40, (*c*) mouth wash, 1 in 480 to 1 in 160, or 1 to 2 ml. in 300 ml.

These agents are specially effective against streptococci. They have the advantage of being non-irritant and non-toxic even in concentrated form. A dilution of 1 in 10 is generally recommended for application to the skin. They may be used as a liquid, ointment or cream.

Chlorhexidine ('Hibitane'). This is an important, non-irritating synthetic disinfectant which remains active in the presence of blood and body fluids and, therefore, has many uses.

It is prepared as a 5% solution or concentrate and also as a powder, obstetric cream (1%), antiseptic cream (1%) and lozenge. It may be mixed with the detergent, cetrimide, to form a very useful cleansing agent.

Hexachlorophane ('Phisohex') may be used for preoperative skin cleansing, routine hand washing and skin care generally. It is of value in the prevention and treatment of staphylococcal infections in the newborn.

When combined with neomycin ('Naseptin') it forms a useful cream for the treatment of nasal carriers of staphylococci.

Dequalinium ('Dequadin') has antiseptic properties and is used in lozenges, pessaries, paint, cream and impregnated gauze.

4. THE HALOGENS

The term halogen (which is derived from two Greek words meaning "salt producer") is used for the elements chlorine, iodine and bromine and fluorine because their salts are found in seawater. The disinfectant drugs of this group owe their germicidal power to the liberation of chlorine or iodine in small quantities.

Chlorine itself is a poisonous, intensely irritating, green gas which has no medicinal use in this form. The following compounds are, however, employed:

Chlorinated lime or bleaching powder (*Calx chlorinata*).

Hypochlorite solutions, which include Eusol, and 'Milton'.

The chloramines.

Chlorinated lime or bleaching powder is a disinfectant and deodorant of special use in disinfecting faeces, deodorizing drains and lavatories, and is the basis of other preparations.

Eusol (*Liquor calcis chlorinatae cum acido borico*) is a solution of chlorinated lime and boric acid which is used for the irrigation and dressing of wounds. It is non-irritating and non-toxic. Solutions tend to decompose on keeping and should not be more than three weeks old. Dressings are applied in the form of gauze soaked in Eusol and should not be covered with waterproof material.

'Milton' is a pleasant proprietary preparation having sodium hypochlorite as a base which may be used for cleaning and irrigating wounds, as a dressing and for storing dentures and babies' feeding bottles.

Chloramine is a complicated organic compound containing chlorine and has similar uses to the former preparations.

Chlorine preparations are also used in the disinfection of drinking water and the water in public swimming baths. The unpleasant taste of the water may be neutralized by the addition of sodium thiosulphate (photographic "hypo") after the chlorine has been permitted to act for a definite period.

Iodine (*Iodum*)

Iodine is an element which is in the form of bluish-black crystals. It is intensely irritating to the skin, which it stains a deep reddish brown. This may be removed by solutions of alkali or sodium thiosulphate.

In addition to its antiseptic properties, iodine and its salts have many other uses in medicine.

The disinfectant preparation most commonly employed is tincture of iodine (*Liquor iodi mitis*, B.P.—Weak solution of iodine, $2\frac{1}{2}$ per cent). This is an alcoholic solution which must be distinguished from *Liquor iodi aquosus*, B.P.C., sometimes known as Lugol's solution. The latter is used for internal administration, especially in cases of thyrotoxicosis before operation, in doses increasing from 0·3 to 1 ml. (2 to 15 minims), (see also p. 197).

Tincture of iodine is employed as a skin disinfectant and sometimes as a vaginal douche (4 ml. in 500 ml., 60 minims to a pint). Preparations: (a) for external use.

Strong solution of iodine (*Liquor iodi fortis*).

Weak solution, or tincture, of iodine (*Liquor iodi mitis*).

Compound iodine paint, or Mandl's paint (*Pigmentum iodi compositum*). (Sometimes used for sore throats.)

Iodine ointment (*Unguentum iodi*).

Povidone–iodine ('Betadine') solution and ointment.

(b) for internal use.

Aqueous solution of iodine and potassium iodide or Lugol's solution (*Liquor iodi aquosus*).

Radio-active iodine (^{131}I and ^{132}I) are used in the diagnosis and treatment of disorders of the thyroid gland.

Iodine compounds for X-ray diagnosis

There are a number of substances containing iodine which are opaque to X-rays and which can be introduced into the body without causing harm. They can be used for outlining the bronchial tree (bronchogram), the uterus (uterogram or hysterogram), the fallopian tubes (salpingogram), the spinal cord (myelogram), the gall bladder (cholecystogram), the urinary tract (pyelogram).

In the case of the cholecystogram the dye is usually taken by mouth and is excreted by the liver so that normally it fills the gall bladder. A pyelogram may be obtained by injecting the dye intravenously.

These compounds include:

1. Propyliodone ('Dionosyl') which is used for bronchograms.

2. Sodium diatrizoate ('Hypaque'), which is used for intravenous and retrograde pyelograms and also for other radiographic procedures.

3. 'Salpix' and 'Endografin FL', for hystero-salpingography.

4. 76% 'Urografin' or 70% sodium iothalamate ('Conray 420'), for arteriography.

5. 'Myodil' which may be injected intrathecally by means of lumbar puncture.

6. Gall bladder dyes which include sodium ipodate ('Biloptin') 'Solu-Biloptin' and 'Telepaque' which are given by mouth and 'Biligrafin' given intravenously.

Iodoform. This is an organic compound, yellow in colour, with a strong odour which many persons find objectionable. It has the reputation of being an antiseptic, but its value is doubtful. It is sometimes used as a powder for insufflation into the ear. Mixed with bismuth subnitrate in the form of a paste (*Pasta bismuthi et iodoformi*, known also as BIPP), it is sometimes used for packing wounds and sinuses.

Whitehead's varnish (*Pigmentum iodoformi compositum*) may be employed to protect the skin from irritating discharges.

N.B.—Some individuals are sensitive to iodine in any form. Toxic effects such as flushing, nausea, vomiting, skin eruptions and, rarely, collapse may be observed.

Fluorine. This element is present in natural water supplies and in places where the drinking water contains fluoride in a concentration of one part per million the incidence of dental caries (tooth decay) is strikingly low. In areas where the water supplies lack fluoride, the level can be artificially increased to 1 p.p.m., a process called fluoridation. In areas where this has been done, the incidence of caries has fallen to a level similar to that in areas where fluoride occurs naturally in the water at a similar concentration. The substances used to fluoridate water are sodium fluoride and sodium silicofluoride. Fluoride is incorporated into the enamel of teeth and protects it against attack by acids. It is also incorporated into the film (plaque) which normally covers teeth. This film contains bacteria which break down carbohydrate to acids which attack teeth. Fluoride inhibits the bacterial enzymes responsible for this breakdown.

Sodium fluoride in a dose of 40 mg three times per day may be used to strengthen bone in myelomatosis.

5. OXIDIZING AGENTS

The most important drugs which owe their antiseptic properties to the liberation of oxygen in the presence of organic matter are hydrogen peroxide and potassium permanganate.

Hydrogen peroxide (*Hydrogenii peroxidum*, H_2O_2)

This is used in the form of a solution (*Liquor hydrogenii peroxidi*) which contains about 3 per cent of hydrogen peroxide but is described as "10 volumes". This means that it can liberate 10 times its volume of oxygen, and a stronger solution of double this strength is described as being of "20 volumes".

In the presence of organic matter or pus, bubbles of oxygen are liberated, and this has a valuable mechanical action in removing discharges from wounds in addition to its antiseptic property. It must be used with care in the irrigation of deep cavities, especially the thorax, and there must be a free outlet for drainage since the oxygen liberated may produce dangerous distension unless it can escape.

Hydrogen peroxide is used as a mouth-wash and has a slightly bitter taste. After its use as ear-drops the meatus should be carefully dried by swabbing or its epithelium will become sodden. It also acts as an astringent and is a good haemostatic. It is used for bleaching fabrics and the hair, the latter being turned an easily recognizable, un-natural yellow colour not comparable in beauty with that of the natural blonde. It forms the basis of 'Sanitas'.

Potassium permanganate (*Potassii permanganas*)

This occurs in the form of dark purple crystals. It is a disinfectant and deodorant and owes its power to the fact that in solution it gives off oxygen in the presence of organic matter. As it does so it turns brown, an indication that the solution has lost its efficiency. Permanganates form the basis of Condy's Fluid.

It is used in strengths of 1 in 5000 for application to wounds, ulcers, fungus infections etc., and 1 in 10,000 as a vaginal douche, gargle and mouth-wash. The solid is sometimes applied to snakebites but is no longer recommended. Permanganate stains in fabrics may be removed by applying sulphurous acid and then washing in water.

Preparations:

Solutions of potassium permanganate (*Liquor potassii permanganatis*) weak (1 in 8000), strong (1 in 2500).

6. DYES

The most important germicidal dyes can be divided into two main groups which may be conveniently called (*a*) the aniline group and (*b*) the flavine group, thereby indicating their general chemical type.

(a) Dyes of the aniline group

Their main use is in disinfecting the skin and in the antiseptic treatment of wounds. Their action is relatively slow and, as has already been pointed out, is selective in character; that is, they only have a marked effect on certain organisms.

The most important dyes of this group are **crystal violet**, **magenta** and **brilliant green**. The green and violet dyes are sometimes used in

46 *Disinfectants and antiseptics*

combination in the form of Bonney's blue (*Liquor tinctorium*). They are most effective against staphylococci and are more useful in preventing infection than in the treatment of established sepsis, although they are of value in some cases of impetigo. Solutions may be either aqueous or spirituous. For application to the skin a 1 per cent solution is employed; for wounds, dilutions of 1 in 1000 to 1 in 2000 are used.

With acriflavine, they form the basis of triple dye jelly which may be used as a tanning compound in the treatment of small burns.

Crystal (gentian) violet capsules have been given internally for the treatment of thread worms.

Other dyes of this group employed for different purposes include:

Congo red.	Methylene blue.
Indigo carmine.	Scarlet red.

Indigo carmine, when given by intramuscular injection, is excreted by the kidneys and may be used as a test of renal efficiency. The principle is to observe the rate at which the dye is excreted from each kidney after ureteric catheterization.

Methylene blue is also used to test renal efficiency.

(b) **Dyes of the flavine (acridine) group**

These dyes are yellow in colour and show marked selective action against streptococci. The three most commonly used are **acriflavine, proflavine** and **acramine red.** They are used both for application to the skin and for irrigating wounds. As distinct from many other germicides, their action is not decreased by the presence of blood and they do not interfere with the phagocytic power of the leucocytes. They are generally employed in strengths of 1 in 1000, but they must not be mixed with Eusol, lysol or mercurial solutions. Stains are removed with dilute hydrochloric acid.

Emulsions in liquid paraffin are sometimes used, but their antiseptic power is thereby considerably reduced.

7. OTHER SUBSTANCES

Among the other disinfectants which have not so far been mentioned, the most important is formaldehyde.

Formaldehyde (*Formaldehydum*)

Formaldehyde itself is a pungent gas which irritates the eyes and mucous membranes of the respiratory tract. It is used in the form of a solution, *Liquor formaldehydi* (formalin), which contains about

40 per cent of the pure substance. This is a powerful disinfectant but, in a solution of this strength, is unsuitable for application to the skin. It is useful for spraying the walls and furniture of infected rooms, and special fumigators for the liberation of the gas are employed to fumigate rooms. The room is sealed for 3 to 4 hours.

Formaldehyde has an important use in the sterilization of catheters which are exposed in a special box to its vapour. The vapour is obtained either from *Liquor formaldehydi* or from tablets of paraform.

Gas sterilization

Special automatic gas sterilizers using ethylene oxide are available. They are useful for disinfecting mattresses, pillows, clothing and apparatus which might be damaged by other methods. Electronic cardiac pacemakers are sterilized in ethylene oxide gas.

In conclusion, the utmost care must be taken in the use of antiseptics and disinfectants. When employed they must be used in the appropriate strength and allowed to act for the correct time. So many are available that no one can be expected to know the details of all, but it should be regarded as a duty to be familiar with those in common use.

Although these substances are valuable, remember that unless correctly used they can afford a very dangerous false sense of security. Do not imagine for one moment that dipping the hands in a bowl of highly coloured liquid (reputed to be an antiseptic but probably inactive in the dilution employed) by the side of the typhoid or other infectious patient has any other value than to remind you to go and wash your hands at once, and properly, with soap and water. In any case, you should have been wearing rubber or disposable gloves!

Deodorants

Deodorants or deodorizers may be defined as substances which are used to destroy or remove disagreeable odours. Many of them are also disinfectants or antiseptics and have been mentioned in this connection. They may be used to get rid of odours from drains or from offensive discharges from wounds. For the former purpose, chlorinated lime and Jeyes' Fluid are examples of the most economical.

For wounds, hydrogen peroxide, 'Sanitas', Eusol and potassium permanganate are all useful or charcoal may be applied as a powder.

Agents of the lysol and phenol types act as deodorants. Offensive smells can also to some extent be covered by the pungent odour of iodoform or by the burning of special deodorizing cones.

Special electrical apparatus which produces ozone is an efficient method of deodorizing a room. An 'Airwick' is also useful.

A number of deodorant sprays with fancy names are available which, by their own potency, effectively mask unpleasant odours.

Chlorophyll tablets taken by mouth are optimistically claimed to deodorize the breath.

Cetrimide ('Cetavlon') is a detergent which also has antiseptic properties p. 53.

CHAPTER 5

Drugs Acting on the Surface of the Body

There are a number of specialized forms of treatment which are used in various skin and other conditions and also for the relief of superficial pain viz.:

Radiation: X-rays, radium, ultra-violet light

Heat: (a) cautery

(b) radiant heat, infra-red rays

Cold: (a) carbon dioxide snow (for warts and naevi)

(b) evaporating lotions

In addition, medicaments may be employed by local application in various forms including:

Lotions and liniments.

Ointments, creams and pastes.

Paints, powders and poultices.

In order that the above may be applied to the skin a number of different bases or vehicles are employed to incorporate the medicaments used. These include:

1. *Dusting powders* consisting either of unmixed powdered drugs or containing starch, which absorbs moisture, or talc or Fuller's earth which do not.

2. *Water:* (a) Soluble substances may be dissolved in water and applied in various strengths which are usually expressed as a percentage solution.

(b) "Shake lotions", such as calamine lotion, in which the substance does not dissolve but after application the water evaporates leaving the dried medicament in powder form on the skin surface.

3. *Alcohol:* This is included in some lotions for the cooling effect which occurs with rapid evaporation. It is also used as a vehicle in some solutions, liniments and paints, e.g. tincture of iodine which has an antiseptic action.

4. *Water-soluble vehicles and emulsifying agents:* These are non-oily substances of complicated chemical structure (including glycols

and stearates) which produce emulsions from which medicaments are easily absorbed. They include macrogols and substances such as lanette wax which assist in the mixture of watery and oily substances.

5. *Oily and greasy vehicles.* These include soft and hard paraffin, also wool fat and the wood alcohols derived from it. They form the basis of ointments.

The majority of drugs used can be classified according to their main actions:

Antiseptic applications

Some of the antiseptic or bacteriocidal substances already mentioned in the previous chapters are suitable for external application in the form of lotions, paints or creams etc. Among them are:

Salicylic acid.

Formaldehyde (3%) lotion.

Copper and zinc sulphate lotion (astringent and mildly antiseptic).

Brilliant green, magenta and crystal violet paints.

Cetrimide cream.

Chlortetracycline cream.

Proflavine cream.

Chlorhexidine ('Hibitane') cream.

Hexachlorophane ('Phisohex') cream.

Ointments containing penicillin, streptomycin or sulphonamides carry a high risk of causing sensitization and are, therefore, contraindicated as local applications. Tetracycline, chloramphenicol and neomycin are less risky. Impetigo and local skin fissures are the types of condition treated in this way.

Antiparasitic preparations

These include benzyl benzoate application used in the treatment of scabies. Crotamiton cream may also be used in this condition. Sulphur ointment, although effective, is liable to cause further dermatitis.

Gamma benzene application ('Lorexane'), medicated lethane oil and dicophane application are used for pediculosis of the head. Dicophane or 'DDT' (dichlor-diphenyl-trichlorethane) is an insecticide which has many medical and domestic uses but lice may become resistant to it. Other insecticides, e.g. carboryl, are under trial.

Fungicides. There are numerous fungus infections of the skin, hair and nails, including ringworm and monilia infections. Local applications used in treatment of conditions such as "athlete's foot" include magenta paint, benzoic acid compound (Whitfield's) ointment and zinc undecenoate ointment. Proprietary preparations include 'Mycil' (chlorphenesin), 'Asterol', 'Tinaderm' (tolnaftate).

Griseofulvin is an oral antibiotic used in ringworm and certain other fungus infections. The average adult dose is 1 gram daily for three to ten weeks. Finger-nail infections may require longer treatment, up to six months.

Antipruritics

Itching may be a symptom both of skin disorders and general disease such as diabetes, jaundice, drug intoxication and anxiety states. Lotions and creams such as phenol, calamine and crotamiton ('Eurax') have a local action. Antihistamine drugs by mouth may be helpful but when applied locally may cause sensitization.

Local steroid preparations such as hydrocortisone and prednisolone lotions and creams (up to 1 per cent) are valuable and may be combined with antibiotics such as tetracycline in infective skin lesions.

Caustics (Escharotics)

A caustic is a substance which has a burning or destructive action on living tissue. Many concentrated disinfectants are caustics and have been mentioned already. They include:

Strong nitric, hydrochloric and sulphuric acids.

Glacial acetic acid and trichloracetic acid.

Chromic acid.

Acid mercuric nitrate.

Silver nitrate, copper sulphate and zinc chloride.

Caustic potash and caustic soda.

Strong acids are sometimes used to destroy warts.

Silver nitrate is used to burn down excess of granulation tissue in a healing wound, in order that the epithelium may have an opportunity of growing over the surface of the granulation tissue from the sides of the wound. Silver nitrate may be applied to dog bites.

Copper sulphate is applied to the inner surface of the eyelids in trachoma.

Acid mercury nitrate in solution, has been applied to the skin lesions in lupus vulgaris.

Chromic acid, 25 per cent, is sometimes applied as a cauterizing agent to the septum of the nose to stop haemorrhage from a bleeding-point in severe epistaxis.

Emollients

Emollients are bland oily substances applied to the skin or mucous membranes to protect them from irritation or to render them soft. They are therefore useful in the treatment of abrasions, chapped hands and healing surfaces. They also serve as vehicles for other drugs applied for various diseases in the form of ointments. (Not all ointments, however, are emollient in action.) The most important emollients are:

Wool fat and 'Lanolin'.   Soft paraffin ('Vaseline').
Olive oil.   Castor oil.
Arachis oil.

Barrier creams are preparations designed to protect the skin against irritant substances which may be encountered by industrial workers or nurses. They may also be used to protect the skin of patients from discharges. Silicone barrier creams are water-repellent and are used against water-soluble irritants. They are useful in the prevention of napkin rash and in the treatment of bed sores.

Demulcents

These are substances similar to emollients which are applied to mucous membranes and may be given internally. They are used:

For protecting inflamed mucous surfaces, e.g. white of egg or milk given in corrosive poisoning.

Masking the unpleasant taste of certain drugs.

Suspending insoluble drugs.

In addition to the above emollient drugs, gelatin, starch, gum and tragacanth are all demulcents.

Sedative applications

When the skin is acutely inflamed wet dressings are often indicated. These include aluminium acetate lotion, coal tar lotion, lead lotion, calamine lotion and sodium chloride solution (normal saline).

Starch poultices are useful for removing crusts such as may occur in severe impetigo of the scalp.

Soaps

Soaps are cleansing agents made by combining oils or fats with alkalis. There are three main types:

Curd or animal soap made from animal fat and caustic soda.

Hard soap made from vegetable oils and caustic soda.

Soft soap made from vegetable oils and caustic soda or potash but containing glycerin. Ether soap is a 40% solution of soft soap in alcohol and ether.

Soapless washing powders for domestic use are special (sulphonated) fatty alcohols. An example of this type of compound used medicinally is *Liquor sulphestolis* ('Teepol') which is employed as a skin cleanser and shampoo.

Detergents and cleansing agents

These are cleansing agents for the skin. In addition to the use of ordinary soap and water, ether soap, spirit soap or a detergent when the skin is grimed with oil, it may be necessary to remove dirt or crusts from injured or inflamed skin by using olive-oil, arachis oil or starch poultices.

Detergents are more effective cleansing agents than soap and water and in addition many have mild antiseptic properties. Among the most important are:

Cetrimide ('Cetavlon', CTAB which is generally used as a 1% solution. A cream is also available. Napkins may be washed in 1 in a 1000 solution to prevent napkin rash.

Benzalkonium chloride ('Roccal', 'Zephiran') has similar properties. Various strengths are employed according to the particular requirements.

A number of household detergents and washing powders are in use and are well advertised! These occasionally cause dermatitis in persons with a sensitive skin. Care should always be taken not to employ them in concentrated form, and always to rinse the hands well after use.

Astringents

These are drugs which check secretion and cause drying of a surface. They are most frequently used on mucous membranes and, therefore, in addition to their application to the mouth and throat, they are also given internally for their action on the bowel, especially in the treatment of diarrhoea.

Calamine lotion and lead lotion have a slightly astringent action and are used in the acute stages of eczema and also to allay irritation in urticaria. Calamine liniment, various creams (e.g. ichthammol), and Lassar's paste are used in the later stages of eczema. Coal-tar preparations have mildly astringent and antiseptic properties.

Other powerful astringents for external use include tannic acid, alum, iron perchloride and weak solutions of silver nitrate and zinc sulphate.

Stimulating preparations

In order to stimulate the growth of granulation tissue in healing wounds, Red lotion (*Lotio rubra*, containing zinc sulphate) or Scarlet red ointment (*Unguentum rubrum*, containing scarlet red dye) may be applied. Cod-liver oil applied externally has similar properties. Preparations used on the unbroken skin, include ichthammol ointment, zinc and coal tar paste.

Softening preparations (Keratolytics)

It is sometimes necessary to soften the horny layers of the skin, and for this purpose pastes or ointments containing resorcin or salicylic acid may be used.

Chrysarobin is used for removing the scales of psoriasis.

Dithranol has a similar action.

Stains produced by these substances may be removed with a solution of chlorinated lime.

Salicylic acid collodion is used in the treatment of corns.

Irritants

Depending upon the severity of their action, irritants may be classified as:

1. Rubifacients.   2. Vesicants.   3. Caustics (p. 51).

Rubifacients are drugs used to produce reddening or mild inflammation of the skin. By their action they cause the blood vessels to dilate so that the part to which they are applied becomes red and hot. For example, ammonia, camphor, menthol, oil of wintergreen (methyl salicylate), turpentine, all of which are employed in the form of liniments. Kaolin poultice also has a rubifacient action. It is mainly used for the relief of pain, e.g. pleurisy.

Vesicants or blistering agents produce an intense irritation resulting in the formation of blisters. They are no longer used, but include croton oil and cantharides (*Liquor epispasticus* contains cantharidin which is a most violent poison).

Counter-irritation. Remedies such as the liniments, plasters, poultices and paints already referred to, applied to the surface of the body with the object of relieving pain or congestion in an underlying organ by producing mild inflammation of the skin are called counter-irritants.

Pain resulting from a diseased organ is often felt in some part of the body wall rather than in the organ itself. As examples, the pain of a gastric ulcer may be felt in the epigastric region of the abdominal wall and is associated with excessive tenderness of the skin (hyperaesthesia) in that area. Pain in gall bladder disease may be felt in the right shoulder.

This phenomenon is called "referred pain" and is due to the fact that the organ affected has a nerve supply from the same segment of the spinal cord as that of the area of skin in which the pain is felt.

Styptics or haemostatics

Drugs which check bleeding

Styptics are drugs applied *locally* to a bleeding surface with the object of checking haemorrhage. They are unlikely to be of marked effect except in oozing or capillary haemorrhage, bleeding from arteries requiring ligature or repair. Most astringents are also styptics,

e.g. Solution of ferric chloride (*Liquor ferri perchloridi*).
Silver nitrate.
Alum.

Hydrogen peroxide has a useful local haemostatic action. Adrenaline (1 in 1000) applied locally acts by causing the blood vessels in the bleeding area to contract. Caustics will stop haemorrhage but are not employed for this purpose.

Snake venom obtained from a viper (e.g. 'Stypven') is a very powerful haemostatic which may be applied on cotton wool in a dilution of 1 in 10,000. It may be used for plugging bleeding tooth sockets and is especially valuable in the control of bleeding in haemophilia.

The application of absorbable **gelatin sponge** to a bleeding surface promotes a clot which forms rapidly and adheres to the tissues. It may be moistened before use with saline and a wound closed over it. Complete absorption takes place in four to six weeks. Oxidized cellulose and calcium alginate are similarly employed and may, if necessary, be soaked in a solution of thrombin before use.

The treatment of haemorrhage is, however, a much wider subject and involves the use of drugs given internally:

1. Morphine is given to allay restlessness and thereby to cause a general lowering of blood pressure.

2. Special haemostatic preparations, e.g.

   'Epsikapron' (aminocaproic acid); used to treat bleeding which is due to fibrinolysis (dissolution of the fibrin in clots).

3. Special drugs such as ergot and ergometrine, and posterior pituitary extract ('Pitocin', p. 212) are given to check bleeding from the pregnant uterus because they have a special action on this organ, causing its muscle to contract.

4. In certain circumstances the tendency to excessive bleeding may be checked by the administration of vitamin K (Menaphthone or phytomenadione) (p. 186). Vitamin K is necessary for the production of prothrombin and is given as a preoperative measure in cases of jaundice. Rutin is a drug used in cases in which increased fragility of the capillaries is present.

Drugs which prevent clotting (anticoagulants)

There are a number of substances which have a directly opposite *local* action to the styptics, namely, they prevent blood from clotting. These include:

1. Sodium and potassium citrates. They act by preventing the activity of the calcium salts present in the blood by combining with them to form inactive compounds. Use is made of this in blood transfusion by collecting blood into 3·8 per cent citrate solution.

2. Sodium oxalate has a similar effect and is used for preventing the clotting of blood taken for certain laboratory tests, e.g. blood

cholesterol, creatinine, urea, uric acid and the Van den Burgh and other liver function tests. Sodium fluoride may be used in blood-sugar estimation.

N.B.—Citrates given internally do not have any effect on the clotting of blood. Oxalates and fluorides are poisonous.

3. Contact with oil, grease or paraffin wax.

4. Hirudin, a substance obtained from the leech, delays clotting. This explains why a leech bite continues to bleed for a considerable period.

5. The anticoagulant drugs given *internally*, including heparin, phenindione ('Dindevan') and nicoumalone ('Sinthrome'), are considered on p. 108.

Diaphoretics

The sweat glands are situated in the skin all over the body but are most abundant in the axillae, palms, soles and forehead, and have been estimated to number about two million. They are supplied by the sympathetic nerves.

Drugs which increase the amount of perspiration are called diaphoretics. They may act:

1. By stimulating the sweating centre in the central nervous system.
2. By stimulating the sweat glands.
3. By dilating the cutaneous blood vessels, which increase the blood supply to the glands.

It is not always possible to say exactly how and where each diaphoretic drug acts. The following are examples of diaphoretics:

Pilocarpine, a very powerful drug, which stimulates the nerves of the involuntary system supplying the sweat glands.

Alcohol, which acts by dilating the cutaneous blood vessels.

Ipecacuanha. This has a mild diaphoretic action and is a constituent of Dover's powder *Pulvis ipecacuanhae et opii*).

The main use of diaphoretics is to render a feverish patient with a hot dry skin more comfortable. The evaporation of the sweat also tends to cause a fall in the body temperature (i.e. diaphoretics have an antipyretic action).

Anhidrotics are drugs which diminish the amount of sweat. The most important are atropine and belladonna, and stramonium. They also cause dryness of the mouth.

Antipyretics

An antipyretic is a drug which reduces fever. There are a number of antipyretic drugs, but all have other actions for which they are employed, so that their antipyretic effect is incidental to their use for other purposes.

C

The normal temperature of the body is maintained by a balance between the heat produced and the heat lost, and this is controlled by the heat-regulating centre in the brain. Heat lost is dependent on (*a*) the amount of blood circulating in the vessels of the skin and (*b*) the amount of sweat secreted and the rate of evaporation.

A drug may therefore have an antipyretic effect:

  (i) by acting on the heat-regulating centre,
 (ii) by dilating the blood vessels in the skin,
(iii) by increasing the amount of sweat.

The drugs which have an antipyretic action include:

Aspirin and sodium salicylate.   Quinine.   All diaphoretics.

The methods employed when it is desired to lower body temperature are tepid or cold sponging, a tepid bath, etc., details of which are given in books on Nursing.

CHAPTER 6
Drugs Acting on the Alimentary System

DRUGS ACTING ON THE MOUTH AND PHARYNX

Drugs used for their action on the mouth and pharynx are most commonly employed in the form of mouth washes, gargles, paints or lozenges, which may be demulcent, astringent, antiseptic or sedative in character, e.g.

Demulcent: Glycerin.
Glycerin of borax (*Glycerinum boracis*).
(Bioral).
Astringent: Glycerin of tannic acid.
Solution of iron perchloride (*Liquor ferri perchloridi*).
Antiseptic: Phenol (0·5 per cent).
Hydrogen peroxide.
Glycerin of thymol (as in 'Glycothymoline' and *Collutorium thymolis composita*).
Crystal violet paint.
Mandl's paint (*Pigmentum iodi compositum*).
Lozenges, e.g. 'Dequadin', 'Bradosol', 'Tyrozets'.
Sedative: Benzocaine lozenge (*Trochisci benzocainoe compositi*).
Phenol or aspirin gargles, which have an anaesthetic effect.
'Bonjela'
Steroid: Hydrocortisone tablets ('Corlan') for ulcers in the mouth.

These are generally used in various forms of stomatitis, pharyngitis and tonsillitis.

DRUGS ACTING ON THE SALIVARY GLANDS

Drugs may be given either to increase (sialagogues) or decrease (anti-sialagogues) the flow of saliva. Drugs may also decrease the

flow of saliva and cause dryness of the mouth when given for other purposes. Thus atropine reduces the amount of saliva and this may be a troublesome side-effect of its administration.

Hyoscine and stramonium formerly used in large doses in the treatment of paralysis agitans, also produce excessive dryness of the mouth which may be counteracted by giving pilocarpine, a drug which stimulates the flow of saliva.

Sialagogues (increasing flow): pilocarpine.
Anti-sialagogues (decreasing flow): atropine, hyoscine, stramonium.

DRUGS ACTING ON THE TEETH AND GUMS

Toothpastes are generally made of slightly abrasive powders, with soap, to which some antiseptic and a flavouring agent may be added. Fluoride may also be added to help to prevent caries.

Toothache due to dental caries may be relieved by inserting into the cavity a pledget of cotton wool soaked in oil of cloves or 'Dentalone', which have a local anaesthetic action.

Various astringents, crystal violet or weak solution of iodine may be applied to the gums in cases of gingivitis.

DRUGS ACTING ON THE STOMACH

In order to understand the various actions of drugs on the stomach it is important to recall the main points concerning its physiology.

1. The stomach is a hollow organ consisting of serous, muscular and mucous coats. The muscular coat (having circular, longitudinal and oblique fibres) gives it the power of peristaltic movement. The circular fibres also form the pyloric sphincter which relaxes at intervals to allow partially digested food to enter the duodenum.

The glands of the mucous membrane secrete pepsin, which converts proteins into peptones; hydrochloric acid which acts as an antiseptic barrier and aids the action of pepsin; also rennin and the intrinsic factor essential for the absorption of vitamin B_{12}.

Hydrochloric acid may be absent (achlorhydria), diminished (hypochlorhydria) or increased (hyperchlorhydria).

The nerve supply of the stomach includes nerves passing to the vomiting centre in the medulla, which is also connected to the higher centres of the brain.

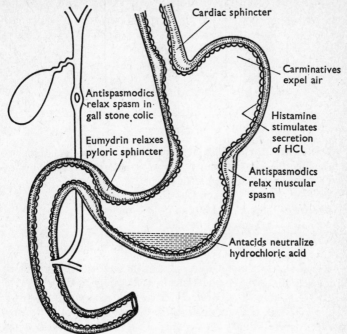

Cardiac sphincter

Carminatives expel air

Antispasmodics relax spasm in gall stone colic

Histamine stimulates secretion of HCl

Eumydrin relaxes pyloric sphincter

Antispasmodics relax muscular spasm

Antacids neutralize hydrochloric acid

FIG. 1.—Diagram illustrating the action of some drugs on the stomach, etc.

Drugs acting on the stomach can be considered according to whether they act (*a*) on its movements or (*b*) on the mucous membrane or its secretions, viz.:

1. Carminatives.
2. Emetics. } Acting on stomach movements.
3. Sedatives and anti-emetics.
4. Stomachics, including bitters—acting on the mucous membrane.
5. Antacids.
6. Substitutes.
7. Drugs used in radiography.

I CARMINATIVES

A carminative is a drug which aids the expulsion of wind from the stomach by increasing the tone of its muscle and stimulating its movements, e.g.

(i) The volatile oils such as oil of peppermint (*Oleum menthae piperitae*) 0·2 ml. ($\frac{1}{2}$ to 3 minims).

(ii) Aromatic spirit of ammonia (*Spiritus ammonii aromaticus* or Sal volatile) 4 ml. (15 to 60 minims) in water.

(iii) Various preparations of ginger (*Zinziber*).

II EMETICS

Emetics are drugs which produce vomiting and are therefore responsible for causing much more violent movements in the stomach muscle than carminatives.

Emetics acting directly on the stomach include:

Tincture of ipecacuanha 30 ml. ($\frac{1}{2}$ to 1 ounce).

Zinc sulphate, 2 grams (10 to 30 grains).

Salt and water

Mustard and water $\Big\}$ 8 grams (120 grains) in 200 ml. of water.

An emetic acting directly on the vomiting centre is apomorphine 6 mg ($\frac{1}{10}$ grain) given hypodermically, but rarely used.

N.B.—Excessive doses of many drugs will cause vomiting, and it is common after the administration of sulphonamides and nitrofurantoin, and in digitalis poisoning. In a number of persons the usual doses of morphine appear to stimulate the vomiting centre.

Emetic drugs are not often employed, as in most cases in which it is desired to empty the stomach of its contents it is preferable to wash it out with water or saline after passing a stomach tube. In some circumstances, however, it may be necessary to use them. They may be employed to remove the contents of the stomach when it is over-distended with food. They are of value, as an emergency measure, in some cases of poisoning due to substances other than caustics, e.g. Ipecacuanha as an alternative to gastric lavage in the emergency treatment of accidental poisoning in children. There is danger in using them after caustic poisoning because the violent contraction of the organ may cause rupture of its walls if they are severely damaged by the corrosive substance.

In order to appreciate their mode of action it is necessary to recall the physiological mechanism of vomiting.

There is a special vomiting centre in the medulla to which pass afferent (sensory) nerves from the stomach and other abdominal viscera. From the centre the efferent (motor) nerves are distributed to the muscle of the stomach, the diaphragm and the muscles of the abdominal wall, which take part in the muscular effort associated with vomiting. There is, therefore, a reflex arc through the vomiting centre from the sensory organ (the mucous membrane of the stomach) to the motor organs just mentioned. The centre is also

The Mechanism of Vomiting

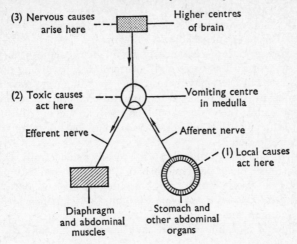

Fig. 2.—Illustrating the mechanism of vomiting.

connected to the higher centres of the brain, including those of sight and smell.

The causes of vomiting

The main causes of vomiting may be listed under the following headings:

1. Peripheral, i.e. local or reflex irritation of the pharynx, stomach or other parts of the alimentary system by stimuli which pass to the vomiting centre.

2. Central

(i) drugs and toxins acting on the centre

(ii) stimuli acting on the higher centres of the brain, e.g.

(a) psychological and emotional factors such as revolting sights and smells, and anxiety states.

(b) organic brain disease (cerebral tumour, meningitis, concussion)

(c) Sea or motion sickness, due to impulses from the labyrinth. Migraine.

SEDATIVES AND ANTI-EMETICS

These are drugs which either tend to diminish the movements of the stomach or else to depress the vomiting centre. They include:

(a)   Drugs of the antihistamine type viz:

      Promethazine ('Avomine')
      Cyclizine ('Marzine')
      Dimenhydrinate ('Dramamine')
      Meclozine ('Ancolan')
} 25–50 mg

(b)   Drugs of the promazine group:

Promazine ('Sparine')   } 25–50 mg
Chlorpromazine ('Largactil') } as anti-emetics.
Perphenazine ('Fentazin'), 2–4 mg

The first group are particularly useful in the prevention and treatment of travel sickness and both groups in vomiting due to other causes but they may increase the effect of alcohol. Cyclizine and similar drugs are reported to have caused foetal abnormalities in animals and, therefore, should be used with great caution in early pregnancy. Most of these drugs may be given by intramuscular injection.

(c) Metoclopramide ('Maxolon') acts locally and centrally. It may be given orally or by intramuscular injection in doses of 10 mg.

(d) Simple drugs which may be used include 'Chlorodyne' (*Tinctura chloroformi et morphinae* 0·6 ml. (5–10 minims), atropine and belladonna, and also barbiturates.

Kaolin and morphine mixture may be used, especially if diarrhoea is present.

IV STOMACHICS, INCLUDING BITTERS

These are given with a view to stimulating the appetite and the secretion of gastric juice, thereby improving digestion and aiding the general nutrition, especially during convalescence. They include gentian and nux vomica and act mainly by suggestion.

V ANTACIDS

These drugs are given in order to neutralize hydrochloric acid in cases of gastric and duodenal ulcer or to neutralize its excess in hyperchlorhydria and in the symptomatic treatment of heartburn. The most important are:

Magnesia (magnesium oxide).   Aluminium glycinate.
Magnesium carbonate.   Bismuth carbonate.
Magnesium trisilicate.   Sodium bicarbonate.
Aluminium hydroxide.

Aluminium hydroxide (sometimes used in the form of 'Aludrox') may also be given as a colloidal solution by the continuous drip method through a nasal catheter.

Sodium bicarbonate in the presence of hydrochloric acid liberates carbon dioxide and later stimulates the further secretion of hydrochloric acid, so is unsuitable for use alone as an antacid and may cause alkalosis in excessive dosage.

A number of the above substances may be mixed together to form special antacid powders, e.g.

(i) Magnesium trisilicate   (ii) Magnesium carbonate
    Magnesium carbonate   Calcium carbonate
    Sodium bicarbonate   Bismuth carbonate
    Calcium carbonate

The doses of the majority of these powders and drugs varies between 2 and 4 grams (30–60 grains).

It must be remembered that some of them tend to have a laxative action which, in certain individuals, is sufficient to cause considerable discomfort. Magnesium trisilicate is free from this defect. (N.B.—Mist. Mag. Trisil., N.F., contains only 600 mg (10 grains) of magnesium trisilicate in each 15 ml. ($\frac{1}{2}$ oz.) dose.) Others given in large doses may produce the condition of alkalosis.

Special compressed tablets consisting of various alkalis which are allowed to dissolve slowly in the mouth between the cheek and lower jaw at the rate of two an hour are an effective means of neutralizing the acid of the gastric juice. (e.g. 'Nulacin', 'Gelusil', 'Prodexin.')

Anticholinergic agents diminish the secretion of gastric acid but it is doubtful whether they hasten the healing of peptic ulcers.

Liquorice preparations often heal gastric ulcers and may heal duodenal ulcers. **Sodium carbenoxolone** is used for both. For gastric ulcers it is supplied as a tablet ('Biogastrone') and for duodenal ulcers it is supplied in "positioned-release" capsules ('Duogastrone'), which rupture in the pylorus to release a concentrated solution of the drug into the duodenum. Carbenoxolone is thought to act by increasing the production of adherent mucus, which helps to protect the mucosa. Side-effects include oedema, hypertension and hypokalaemia in some patients. 'Caved-S', which contains liquorice, is said not to have these unfortunate side-effects.

Doses: 'Biogastrone' Initially 2 t.d.s. for 1 week, then 1 t.d.s., after meals.

      'Duogastrone' 1 q.d.s. 15–30 minutes before meals.

      'Caved-S'   2 t.d.s., chewed and swallowed after meals.

VI SUBSTITUTES

Dilute hydrochloric acid (*Acidum hydrochloricum dilutum*, 5 ml., 5 to 60 minims) may be given in water or orange juice with meals in cases of achlorhydria or hypochlorhydria and may be useful in checking the diarrhoea which somtimes accompanies these conditions.

VII DRUGS USED IN RADIOGRAPHY OF THE STOMACH

A suspension of barium sulphate, which is opaque to X-rays, is generally employed. It is swallowed as a "barium meal", which can be followed by radiography in its course through the oesophagus, stomach, small and large intestines. In addition to showing the outline of the organs this also gives information about their rate of emptying. A "barium enema" is given for examination of the rectum and colon.

OTHER DRUGS USED FOR THEIR ACTION ON THE STOMACH

Atropine methonitrate ('Eumydrin')

As its chemical name implies, this drug is a salt of atropine in composition and has similar actions. It is of special value, however, in being less toxic and more effective in the medical treatment of congenital hypertrophic pyloric stenosis than atropine. By its action it helps to relax the hypertrophied pyloric sphincter and to allow the passage of the stomach contents into the duodenum. It is of value also in relieving the spasms of whooping cough. It may be given in the following ways:

(i) 0·12 to 2 ml. of 0·6% alcoholic solution given on the tongue before each feed. This solution is very potent and must be used with great care. The container must be kept tightly closed to prevent evaporation and must not be confused with atropine methonitrate eye drops. It is unsuitable for out-patients.

(ii) 1 to 5 ml. of a 1 in 10,000 aqueous solution, half an hour before each feed. This is continued for some weeks. The solution must be made up fresh every three days.

The test meal

Charcoal biscuits are sometimes given on the night before the test. A residue of charcoal in the resting juice the following morning indicates that the stomach is not emptying properly, i.e. pyloric stenosis.

Histamine

A subcutaneous injection of 0·04 mg per kg of body weight of histamine acid phosphate is given in certain cases to prove the presence of achylia gastrica, in which there is the complete absence of hydrochloric acid from the gastric juice. Hydrochloric acid may be absent from the juice (achlorhydria), although the stomach is still capable of secreting it. In such instances, histamine will stimulate the glands of the gastric mucous membrane to secrete hydrochloric acid and thereby prove that the case is not one of true achylia gastrica. Using this dose of histamine (maximal histamine stimulation), it is essential always to give an antihistamine, e.g. promethazine first, (subcutaneously $\frac{1}{2}$–1 hr) before the histamine). This will prevent the unpleasant and dangerous effects of histamine but will not interfere with its gastric stimulating effect.

Betazole ('Histalog') 0·5 mg per kg of body weight, intramuscularly, may be used instead of histamine and does not need to be "covered" with an antihistamine.

Pentagastrin ('Peptavlon'), is preferably used for testing gastric secretion. It is given subcutaneously in a dose of 6 micrograms per kg body weight or by intravenous infusion at a rate of 0·01 micrograms per kg per minute.

DRUGS ACTING ON THE INTESTINES

1. Those promoting evacuation. (The aperients, injections, enemata and suppositories)
2. Those which lessen movements and spasm. (Sedatives)
3. Antiparasitic
   (a) antiseptics
   (b) anthelmintics

THE APERIENTS

An aperient is a drug employed in medicine to assist the bowel to evacuate its contents and, in the majority of instances, it does so on account of its power of stimulating peristalsis and the movements of the bowel.

It will be recalled that the onward passage of the intestinal contents is due to two main factors: (i) Peristalsis. (ii) The operation of the important gastro-colic reflex. When food is taken into the stomach this causes a reflex relaxation of the ileocaecal valve by which the contents of the lower ileum rapidly enter the caecum and, as a result, the contents of the colon are passed on into the rectum.

The distension of the rectum thus produced give rise to the natural desire to defaecate.

Aperients are sometimes classified according to the intensity of their action thus:

1. Laxatives. These are relatively mild and result in the hastening of peristaltic action without altering the appearance or consistency of the stools. Simple lubricants such as liquid paraffin may also be included in this group.

2. Mild purgatives. These are stronger in action, producing looser and, sometimes, repeated stools.

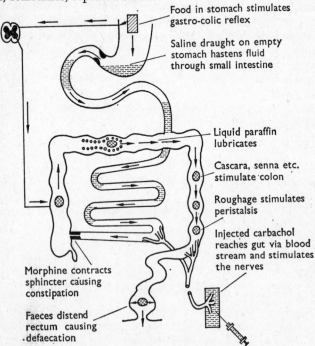

Food in stomach stimulates gastro-colic reflex

Saline draught on empty stomach hastens fluid through small intestine

Liquid paraffin lubricates

Cascara, senna etc. stimulate colon

Roughage stimulates peristalsis

Injected carbachol reaches gut via blood stream and stimulates the nerves

Morphine contracts sphincter causing constipation

Faeces distend rectum causing defaecation

FIG. 3.—Diagram illustrating the action of some aperients.

3. Drastic purgatives. These are violent in action, often accompanied by pain and colic, and resulting in frequent and watery stools comparable with those of acute enteritis.

This classification is to some extent an artificial one because, in a number of instances, the effect produced is dependent upon the dose of the drug administered and, in excessive doses, some of the milder laxatives may act as drastic purgatives. However, from a practical point of view it is useful if the recognized doses of the various drugs are adhered to. The term aperient has here been used to cover all the groups.

Modes of action

Aperients act in various ways.

(i) The principal natural stimulus to peristalsis is the presence of faecal material stretching the muscle of the intestinal wall. Peristalsis is, therefore, more active if the amount of faecal residue is increased. In addition to taking vegetable and cellulose material in the diet to produce "roughage", the bulk of the faeces may be increased by non-absorbable substances, such as agar and 'Isogel', which swell as they take up water present in the gut.

(ii) Certain aperients, particularly those of the saline group, e.g. Epsom salts (magnesium sulphate), act mainly as hypertonic solutions which withdraw fluid via the mucous membrane of the gut. This fluid increases the bulk of the stool. At the same time the increased bulk of the stool causes more rapid peristalsis and, therefore, there is less time for the normal absorption of fluid from the lower bowel.

(iii) Others act by stimulating the nervous mechanism of peristalsis.

(iv) The drastic purgatives produce a definite inflammatory reaction in the mucous membrane of the intestine which results not only in stimulation of peristalsis but also in the outpouring of an inflammatory exudate. This also increases the relative bulk of the intestinal contents and, in addition, the hurried passage of the contents along the gut does not permit time for the normal absorption of fluid mentioned above. Frequent, copious and watery stools are, therefore, obtained.

In some instances the action of the drugs is more marked on the small intestine, in others it is on the large intestine. The main result, however, is to produce a rapid distension of the rectum with the contents of the gut above, which is very similar to the effect of an enema distending the rectum when given from below.

Summary. The effects of aperients are:

1. To increase the active movements of the intestine, i.e. to stimulate peristalsis and to hurry the passage of the intestinal contents.

2. By mild irritation of the intestinal mucous membrane to increase either slightly or greatly the amount of fluid exudate from the mucosa.

3. To hasten the progress of the intestinal contents so that the normal absorption of water by the colon is partially prevented.

4. To produce rapid distension of the rectum and the associated desire to defaecate.

Since the majority of aperients cause mild irritation of the mucous membrane of the gut it should be clear that their habitual use is undesirable. Their constant employment may cause the natural functions of the intestine to become sluggish so that a vicious circle is set up. It is a common experience that individuals who always employ aperients need to take constantly increasing doses of more powerful drugs.

In comparison with acute constipation associated with some temporary disorder or disease, chronic constipation (dyschezia) is, in most instances, due to faulty habits and failure to respond to the natural call to defaecate which occurs when the rectum becomes distended. The ideal treatment of chronic constipation is therefore not the regular administration of aperients but the gradual re-education of the bowel. This can generally be obtained by (a) regular attempts at evacuation assisted by providing an adequate bulk of the faeces in the form of roughage, and (b) simple enemata from the use of which the patient is gradually weaned. (c) Glycerin or bisacodyl ('Dulcolax') suppositories are useful in some cases. Aperients may be of some value at the commencement of the course but should be dropped as soon as possible.

1. Laxatives

Roughage

As already mentioned, the natural stimulus of peristalsis is an adequate bulk of the faeces in the form of food residue consisting mainly of undigested cellulose. Wholemeal bread, vegetables, and fruits, especially figs and prunes, are all of value for this purpose.

Agar

This is prepared from various sea-weeds. It is not altered by digestion but has the power of absorbing water. In so doing it expands considerably in bulk and, by increasing the volume of the faeces, it promotes peristalsis. Agar is sometimes mixed with liquid paraffin to form an emulsion. 'Normacol', 'Isogel', 'Metamucil' and various plant mucilages have a similar action.

Methyl cellulose in the form of granules (e.g. 'Celevac',) helps to retain water and thus adds to the bulk of the stools.

Liquid paraffin

This is a bland mineral oil which passes through the intestinal tract unchanged by the processes of digestion. It has no action on the mucous membrane of the gut, but acts as a simple lubricant, softening the faeces and aiding their passage through the bowel and rectum. There is no advantage in giving excessive doses and, when it appears to "run through" the patient, the dose should be appropriately reduced. The usual dose is 30 ml. ($\frac{1}{2}$ to 1 ounce) at night, or possibly night and morning. Liquid paraffin should never be given to babies because of the risk of aspiration leading to lipoid pneumonia. This complication may also occur in elderly patients, in whom the cough reflex is weakened. Prolonged usage by any patient may lead to deficiency of the fat-soluble vitamins A, D and K by interfering with their absorption. When it is highly emulsified, liquid paraffin may be absorbed to a small extent and may be deposited in the mesenteric lymph nodes where it may cause a chronic inflammatory paraffinoma. It has also been suggested that prolonged use of liquid paraffin may induce cancer of the colon.

Magnesium hydroxide and syrup of figs (*Syrupus ficorum*, 8 ml., 30 to 120 minims) are also laxatives especially useful for children.

2. Mild purgatives

In smaller doses the following drugs will act as laxatives, but in full doses they are mild purgatives.

(a) Saline aperients

The saline aperients act fairly quickly and are best given in warm water on an empty stomach before breakfast.

Sodium sulphate (*Sodii sulphas*, Glauber's salt), 16 grams (30 to 240 grains).

Magnesium sulphate (*Magnesii sulphas*, Epsom salts), 16 grams (30 to 240 grains).

White mixture (*Mistura magnesii sulphatis alba*, BPC), contains magnesium sulphate (4 grams, 60 grains) and light magnesium carbonate (0·6 gram, 10 grains, to 15 ml., $\frac{1}{2}$ ounce) of peppermint water.

Seidlitz powder (*Pulvis effervescens compositus*, B.P.C.) consists of sodium potassium tartrate and sodium bicarbonate in the blue packet and tartaric acid in the white packet. The contents of the blue packet are dissolved in half a pint of cold or warm water; those of the white packet are then added and the draught taken while effervescing.

(b) Drugs of the senna, cascara, rhubarb and aloes group

These are all mild purgatives of vegetable origin which do not produce inflammation of the intestine like the drugs of the drastic purgative group. As a rule they take 10 to 18 hours to produce an effect. Owing to some absorption from the bowel and subsequent excretion in the urine, rhubarb and senna tend to impart to the latter a yellow-brown colour.

Senna may be prepared from the leaflets or pods of the plant. It tends to produce more griping than other members of the group and its main action is on the colon.

Preparations include senna pods, syrup of senna and Black draught, but the effect of these preparations is unpredictable; it may be anything from inert to griping.

A standardized preparation of senna ('Senokot') is available as granules, tablets and syrup. The correct dose is that which gives a comfortable formed motion and it has to be found by individual trial. For adults the dose of granules is usually one to two 5 ml. teaspoonsful. It is possible to "re-educate" the bowel so that the drug can be discontinued. It is a suitable purgative for use in pregnancy but large doses should be avoided.

Cascara sagrada is a bark from which the following important preparations are made:

Cascara sagrada elixir (*Elixir cascarae sagradae*, BP), 4 ml. (30 to 60 minims).

Compound cascara mixture (*Mistura cascarae et belladonnae*, BPC), 10 ml. ($\frac{1}{2}$ ounce).

Compound cascara sagrada tablet (*Tabella cascarae sagradae composita*, BPC), 1 or 2 tablets.

Rhubarb (*Rheum*) is a rhizome from which the following preparations are made: Compound rhubarb pill (*Pilula rhei composita*, BP).

It is also made up as rhubarb and soda mixture (*Mistura rhei composita*, BPC), 10 ml. ($\frac{1}{2}$ ounce).

Aloes is a dried juice obtained from the leaves of aloe plants. Preparations include:

Aloes and nux vomica tablet (*Tab. aloes et nucis vomicae*, BPC), 1 tablet.

Phenolphthalein is a synthetic drug similar in action to the vegetable drugs mentioned above. It is given in doses of up to 300 mg (1 to 5 grains). 'Alophen' pill consists of a mixture of aloes, phenolphthalein, strychnine and belladonna (1 to 3 pills). Belladonna is added to prevent griping.

Bisacodyl ('Dulcolax'), one or two tablets of 5 mg, is a useful and popular aperient also employed as a suppository.

Castor oil (*Oleum ricini*). Applied to the surface of the body, castor oil is a bland substance having an emollient action. It is also used to allay irritation in the eye and, mixed with zinc oxide, as an application to the skin.

In the intestines, however, it is altered in composition by the pancreatic enzymes and substances are produced which have a mildly irritating effect on the intestine, thereby giving the drug its aperient action. It may be given in capsules, as an emulsion, or mixture and various methods have been devised for disguising its taste.

After its aperient action has passed off it tends to have a slightly constipating effect, hence its use in diarrhoea due to poisonous or unsuitable food, when it may be given with a view to emptying the intestine rapidly (2–6 hours) and then checking the condition by its constipating action. It is sometimes given after abdominal operations. Dose up to 30 ml. (1 fluid ounce).

3. Drastic purgatives or cathartics

These drugs are now never employed. They include:
Calomel.   Jalap.   Colocynth.

DRUGS GIVEN BY HYPODERMIC INJECTION

Certain drugs, having an action on the neuro-muscular mechanism of the bowel whereby they increase the tone of the intestinal muscle and stimulate its movements, may be given by hypodermic injection. They are especially useful in postoperative abdominal distension. They include:

Pituitary, posterior lobe injection ('Pituitrin') (0·5 ml.).

Neostigmine injection (0·5 to 2 mg).

Carbachol ('Doryl', 'Moryl') (0·5 mg). The last named are most used and are also employed to stimulate the tone of the stomach muscle in acute dilation of the stomach and to aid expulsion of gas from the colon in intestinal distension and before X-ray examination.

ENEMATA

An enema consists of the injection of fluid into the rectum. Enemas may be given in order to empty the lower bowel, or for other purposes.

The main points to be remembered in the administration of rectal injections are:

(i) Collect all the required apparatus on a tray and cover with a towel before approaching the patient.

(ii) Whenever possible, place the patient in the lateral position. Enemata may be given with the patient on his back or in the knee–elbow position if necessary.

(iii) Do not insert the nozzle of a Higginson's syringe directly into the anus but attach a soft rubber catheter, which may be lubricated with a little 'Vaseline' spread on lint, and inserted into the rectum for two inches. The tube and funnel method is usually employed unless a modern prepacked disposable set is available.

(iv) Fluids should be injected at a temperature of 37°C (98–100°F) unless otherwise prescribed.

(v) After the removal of the catheter the patient should be lifted on to the bed-pan.

Types of enemata

1. Those to be returned (evacuant)
   - Warm water.   Arachis oil.
   - Soap.   Glycerin.
   - Turpentine.   Calcium chloride.

2. Those to be retained.
   - (a) Sedative e.g.   starch and opium.
   - (b) Anaesthetic e.g.   bromethol ('Avertin').
   - (c) Steroid e.g.   prednisolone

The following are the common types of enemata given:

1. Warm water enema.

2. Soap enema (30 mg, 1 oz of soft soap to 500 ml., 20 oz., of warm water).

3. Turpentine enema, 30 ml. (1 oz.) of oil of turpentine is added to the soap enema; or 30 ml. (1 oz.) of oil of turpentine to 360 ml. (12 oz.) of thin starch mucilage. This is especially useful in aiding the removal of flatus and after abdominal operations.

Turpentine has a deleterious effect on rubber and this enema is preferably given with a tube and funnel. If a Higginson's syringe is used it should be cleaned immediately.

4. Calcium chloride, 120 ml. (4 fl. oz.) of 5% solution causes an immediate evacuation and is useful in the management of elderly incontinent patients.

5. Arachis oil enema. Up to 300 ml. (5 to 10 ounces) of arachis oil are warmed in a water bath to 37°C (98°F) and run into the rectum by a tube and funnel. It should be retained from ½ to 1 hour and may be followed in 4 hours by a soap enema if necessary. Olive oil may be used but is more expensive.

6. Glycerin enema. Eight ml. (60 to 120 minims) of glycerin are introduced by means of a catheter attached to a suitable syringe. A glycerin suppository has a similar effect.

7. Sedative enema. This is sometimes given to check excessive diarrhoea. The one employed is the starch and opium enema. For an adult 140 ml. (5 ounces) of thin starch mucilage containing 2·5 ml. (40 minims) of tincture of opium are introduced at a temperature of 38°C (100°F) by the tube-and-funnel method.

(To make thin starch mucilage, take a tablespoonful of starch powder and mix with a little cold water, make this up to 300 ml. (10 oz.) with boiling water and allow to cool.)

Enema rash. Occasionally a patchy erythematous rash develops about 12 hours after an enema has been given. It usually appears on the face, buttocks and knees and may last for 24 hours. It is sometimes mistaken for scarlet fever or measles, but there is no pyrexia, it is not irritating and, as a rule, requires no treatment. Calamine lotion may be applied if desired.

SUPPOSITORIES

Glycerine and bisacodyl ('Dulcolax') are useful evacuant suppositories which are often used instead of enemata. They are valuable for elderly and bed-ridden patients provided the rectum is not full of impacted faeces.

INTESTINAL SEDATIVES

Intestinal sedatives have an opposite action to aperients, for they lessen peristaltic movement and diminish spasm. They are used in enteritis to check diarrhoea, to soothe the mucous membrane and to relieve colic. They may be classified thus:

(a) Soothing agents

Kaolin, chalk, bismuth salts and magnesium trisilicate are

examples of drugs which help to protect the mucous membrane by their soothing action.

Kaolin and charcoal also adsorb intestinal gases and prevent over-distension of the bowel, thus diminishing its movement and the colicky pains which are caused by the distension.

(b) Drugs acting on nervous mechanism

Atropine and belladonna, and morphine and opium all act on the nervous mechanism. Atropine helps to relax spasm, while morphine has a general depressing effect on the muscular movements and tends to produce constipation.

Proprietary preparations which have an antispasmodic action on the alimentary tract include propantheline ('Probanthine'), 'Antrenyl', 'Merbentyl', 'Wyovin', mebeverine ('Colofac'.)

Among the most useful remedies for diarrhoea are mixtures containing kaolin or bismuth salts and a small dose of morphine, e.g. *Mistura Kaolin et Morphinae* (p. 146); and Chlorodyne (p. 64). Codein phosphate (60 mg, 1 gr.) or diphenoxylate ('Lomotil') are of value. For infective cases sulphonamides or antibiotics are often employed.

(c) Drugs acting on rectum and anus

These are usually in the form of suppositories or ointments which have an astringent or local anaesthetic action, e.g. Bismuth subgallate suppository,

Hamamelidis ointment and suppository,

Benzocaine ointment,

Hydrocortisone suppository.

Diarrhoea associated with achlorhydria sometimes responds to the administration of hydrochloric acid (p. 65).

ANTIPARASITIC DRUGS

(a) Intestinal antiseptics.

(b) Anthelmintics.

1. Intestinal antiseptics

Under normal circumstances the presence of hydrochloric acid in the stomach helps to prevent the growth of bacteria, and in health this freedom from living organisms is maintained throughout the upper part of the small intestine. From the lower end of the ileum, however, the number of bacteria present increases and they are very numerous in the colon. Here they play a part in the digestive processes by helping to break down cellulose, which is unaffected by the digestive juices in the stomach and small intestine.

Sometimes bacteria pass through the hydrochloric acid barrier and cause inflammation of the intestine (enteritis and colitis) or special conditions such as typhoid fever, bacillary dysentery and food poisoning. The bacteria which may be found in the intestines may, therefore, be classified as (*a*) pathogenic, or those responsible for disease of the intestines and (*b*) non-pathogenic, that is those organisms which are normally present in the intestines but cause no disease when they are confined to the bowel. They may, however, be harmful if they reach the peritoneum or other tissues. Included in this group are the organisms which assist in the digestion of cellulose in the colon. In certain circumstances these organisms may cause excessive putrefaction of the bowel contents or excessive fermentation, with the production of gas, some of which may be absorbed by kaolin or charcoal.

The usual method of treatment employed in a case of food poisoning or severe diarrhoea is:

(i) To allay the irritation of the mucous membrane by a mixture containing kaolin and morphine.

(ii) To relieve pain and spasm, if necessary, with morphine and atropine.

(iii) To absorb gas and intestinal toxins by charcoal or kaolin.

(iv) To replace the fluid lost from the body by diarrhoea by giving fluids orally, subcutaneously or intravenously, especially in infants.

(v) To avoid further irritation of the bowel by giving a light and easily digested diet commencing with milk, gruel and arrowroot.

(vi) To give one of the sulphonamides or antibiotics by mouth if a definite organism is found to be responsible for the condition.

(vii) In some cases to get rid of the infected material as soon as possible by an aperient, e.g. castor oil, supplemented if necessary by lavage of the colon with normal saline.

Sulphonamides, including the insoluble ones which are not absorbed from the bowel such as sulphaguanidine, 'Sulfasuxidine' and 'Sulfathalidine', affect the growth of intestinal bacteria. A popular preparation is 'Guanimycin' (a mixture of sulphaguanidine and streptomycin). Tetracycline, chloramphenicol, etc., when given by mouth destroy many bacteria in the intestines (p. 240). If given for more than a few days, however, not only do they permit the overgrowth of many bacteria which are insensitive to them but they may also seriously affect the absorption of certain vitamins, particularly those of the vitamin B complex. Preparations of vitamin B must, therefore, be given at the same time if their administration is prolonged. Erythromycin may be valuable in cases of enteritis caused by staphylococci.

Obviously minor degrees of diarrhoea of short duration do not necessarily require any active treatment.

Treatment of special bowel infections

Dysentery. There are two types of dysentery:

(a) Amoebic dysentery caused by a single-celled organism known as the *Entamoeba histolytica*. In addition to general symptomatic treatment (fluid and electrolyte replacement) the following drugs may be employed.

1. Metronidazole ('Flagyl'), 800 mg, t.d.s. for 5 days.

2. A combination of (a) tetracycline, 250 mg, 6 hourly for 10 days.

    (b) diloxamide ('Furamide'), 500 mg, t.d.s. for 10 days;

    (c) chloroquine, after a starting dose of 600 mg, 150 mg, twice daily for 14 days. This helps to protect the liver from infection.

3. Tinctine hydrochloride, 65 mg daily by intramuscular injection for 5 days (approx.) together with tetracycline and 'Furamide'.

(b) Bacillary dysentery. This may be treated with:

(1) Sulphonamides, e.g. trisulphonamide, sulphaguanidine or phthalysulphathiazole.

(2) Antibiotics e.g. tetracycline, streptomycin.

(3) Nalidixic acid, ('Negram') or neomycin. All drugs are given for 5 to 7 days.

2. Anthelmintics

The intestinal canal may become the home of various parasitic worms. The ova or eggs of the parasites usually enter the human being (the host) in contaminated food or water. They reach the intestine, where they mature into the fully grown worm.

Drugs used in the treatment of worms are called **anthelmintics**. Those which actually kill the worm are sometimes referred to as **vermicides** while those which merely cause its expulsion from the body are called **vermifuges**.

The following are the most important varieties of worm found in this country:

Thread worms.   Tape worms.
Round worms.   Hook worms.

Thread worms (*Enterobius vermicularis*), Enterobiasis
These are common in children and inhabit the large intestine. Their successful eradication depends entirely upon the prevention of reinfection. Their presence is often associated with itching of the anus, for which benzocaine ointment may be applied. Other members of the household should also be checked for the presence of worms or ova.

Treatment. Any of the following drugs may be used:

(i) **Viprynium** ('Vanquin') is given as a single dose according to body weight (5 mg per kg). A repeated dose, after two weeks, is advisable. It stains the stools red.

(ii) **Thiabendazole** ('Mintezol'). Dose: 10 mg/lb of body weight twice daily for 1 to 2 days. Maximum daily dose: 3 G. The drug should be taken after food. It is effective not only against threadworm, but also against roundworms and hookworms.

(iii) **Piperazine** e.g. 'Antepar', 'Veroxil', 'Entacyl', 'Pripsen'. Dose (of base): 500–2000 mg, according to body weight, daily for 7 days.

(iv) **Crystal violet** (*Viola crystallina*) given in enteric-coated capsules is effective. The adult dose is 60 mg (1 grain), t.d.s. with meals; for children up to 10 mg ($\frac{1}{6}$ grain) for each year of age. Two courses each lasting eight days with an interval of a week are given.

Round worms (*Ascaris lumbricoides*) Ascariasis
These resemble the earth worm in appearance and, in addition to entering the intestine, may occasionally wander into the stomach from which they may be vomited, or into the bile ducts when they produce jaundice. The larvae may reach the lungs and cause pneumonia.

Treatment. The following drugs are used:

(i) **Piperazine** is the safest drug to use. A single dose of 4 grams may be given to an adult. For children the dose is calculated according to the age and weight. No purgative is necessary unless constipation is present.

(ii) **Bephenium** ('Alcopar') is also an ascaricide. It is useful for mixed hookworm and round worm infections.

(iii) **Dichlorovos** is active against roundworms and whipworms.

(iv) **Tetramisole** ('Nilverin'), better known as a veterinary anthelminthic, is effective against ascaris and enterobius vermicularis infections in man.

Tape worms (*Taenia solium, Taenia saginata*) Taeniasis

The effective treatment of tape worms requires careful adherence to a strict routine. Drugs which may be used include:—

(i) **'Yomesan'** (niclosamide) kills and partially dissolves tape worms. Two tablets (2G) are well chewed and followed by two more one hour later without previous dieting and subsequent purgation.

(ii) **Dichlorophen** ('Anthphen'), 70 mg per kg body weight, may be used against beef tapeworms but not against pork tapeworms. No starvation or purgation is necessary. The worm is partially digested and there is no point in searching the stools for the head after dichlorophen.

(iii) **Male fern.** In order that the anthelmintic drug may come into full contact with the worm, it is necessary for the stomach and intestines to be as empty as possible. The patient is, therefore, starved for 2 days, fluids only being given. Saline aperients are taken each morning. On the third morning Male Fern Extract Draught (BPC), 50 ml., is given and followed 2 hours later by 15 to 30 G of magnesium sulphate. If the bowels are not opened within an hour or so, a soap and water enema is administered.

The motions should be collected in warm water and a search made for the head of the worm. If it is not found the treatment should be repeated in 10 days.

Under no circumstances should castor oil be given after *Filix mas*, as a combination of these drugs produces very dangerous toxic symptoms.

(iv) **Mepacrine hydrochloride.** This drug which is used in the treatment of malaria is also effective against tape worms. 100 mg are given every five minutes for ten doses (total 1 gram). It is often given via a tube directly into the duodenum as vomiting may occur when it is taken by mouth. Its action is less certain than that of male fern.

Hook worms (*Ancylostoma*)

The ova of these worms may be found in the faeces of patients from tropical countries. The larvae bore their way through the skin and reach the duodenum via the blood vessels, lungs and trachea, causing anaemia and eosinophilia. **Bephenium** ('Alcopar'), 5 grams, repeated in one week is used in treatment.

Tetrachlorethylene, 0·1ml./Kg body weight up to 5 ml., may be used, but is more toxic. An overnight fast and a saline purge is required before administration of the drug. Another saline purge is given 1–2 hours after the drug.

Whipworm
Thiabendazole may be tried, also dithiazanine ('Telurid').

Filariasis
Diethylcarbamazine is used but there may be an allergic response.

Schistosomiasis
Niridazole is employed. It is also used for Guinea worms. Hycanthone, given as a single intramuscular injection, is another effective drug.

Trichiniasis
No drugs are very effective but emetine may be tried.

DRUGS ACTING ON THE LIVER AND BILIARY APPARATUS

There are few drugs which can be used to alter the functions of the liver or to increase the formation of bile, but certain substances hasten the evacuation of bile from the gall bladder into the duodenum. They are called *cholagogues* and include:

Sodium salicylate (2 grams, 10 to 30 grains), sodium sulphate (16 grams, 120 to 240 grains) and magnesium sulphate (2–16 grams, 30–240 grains).

Sulphonamides and certain antibiotics (ampicillin and rifamycin) are the most effective biliary antiseptics.

The injection of adrenaline (1 in 1000) causes the liver to convert the glycogen stored in it into glucose, which passes into the blood. This fact is sometimes made use of in the treatment of hypoglycaemia due to overdosage of insulin.

A fatty meal or the administration of olive oil into the stomach or duodenum causes the gall bladder to empty its contents into the duodenum.

Glucose is said to have a "protective" action on the liver and helps to diminish the damage done to the organ in various toxic states. Calcium gluconate is also given for the same purpose but it is difficult to explain their mode of action, if any.

Cholecystography

Phenobutiodil ('Biliodyl'), Ipanoic acid ('Telepaque'), sodium ipodate ('Biloptin') or calcium ipodate ('Solu-Biloptin'), when given by mouth, are absorbed in the alimentary tract and excreted by the liver into the bile. For a time they are stored and concentrated in the gall bladder. These substances are opaque to X-rays and an X-ray picture can therefore be obtained showing the outline of the gall bladder, provided it is functioning normally.

Technique. On the day before the examination is carried out, the amount of fat in the diet is reduced to a minimum. The patient has a light supper containing no fat at 7 p.m. At 10 p.m. 3 grms of the dye dissolved in water are given, followed by further drinks of water. X-ray pictures are taken next morning. Often, a second dose of the contrast medium is given 2–3 hours before the X-ray examination. During this period no food is allowed, but water may be drunk. The first meal is given one hour before the last X-ray. This consists of a fatty meal which should contain bread, butter, bacon and a cup of tea. Alternatively a fat emulsion containing nut oil ('Prosparol'), dose: 120 ml., 4 fl. oz., may be used.

The gall bladder may not be visualized in some cases, such as when pyloric stenosis or conditions causing diarrhoea interfere with absorption of the dye. Seriously impaired liver function and inability of the diseased gall bladder to concentrate dye are other reasons for failure to visualize the gall bladder. Except in the case of seriously impaired liver function, the gall bladder may be outlined by dye injected intravenously. Iodipamide ('Biligrafin') is used for this purpose and for visualizing the common bile duct; 20 ml. of a 30% solution or of a 50% solution ('Biligrafin forte') are injected intravenously over the course of ten minutes.

PANCREAS

Strong Pancreatin powder is used in cases of malabsorption due to disease of the pancreas, e.g. fibrocystic disease. It may be sprinkled on food or given in a liquid with each meal. The dose varies with the age of the child (up to 1 year, 0·5 to 1 G; 1 to 12 years, 1 to 2 G).

CHAPTER 7

The Action of Drugs on the Heart and Circulation

In order to understand the action of drugs on the heart and circulatory system it is necessary to review certain aspects of their physiology.

1. The heart muscle acts as a pump which supplies the motive force, driving the blood under pressure through the arterial system to all the organs and tissues of the body where it is distributed in the capillaries. The veins are the "return" channels of the circulatory system.

The volume of blood passing through the heart each minute is called the cardiac output. In health cardiac output varies according to the immediate needs of the body, being increased on exercise by an increase in the rate and force with which the heart beats.

In cardiac failure, when the myocardium can no longer supply sufficient force, the cardiac output is reduced. This leads to:

(i) Inadequate blood supply to the organs and tissues.

(ii) Diminished activity of the kidneys causing salt and water retention and oedema.

(iii) Venous congestion.

2. In order to act efficiently the muscle must be adequately nourished. In particular, it requires oxygen and glucose to satisfy its metabolic needs. These reach it in the blood supplied to it through the coronary arteries. Diminution in the size of the lumen of the coronary arteries, either temporarily as a result of spasm or permanently owing to disease of their walls, will result in defective nutrition of the heart muscle, with either temporary or permanent effects on its efficiency.

3. The pressure of blood within the arteries is dependent on (i) the force of the heart beat, i.e. the strength of the muscular contraction, (ii) the calibre of the arteries, (iii) the elasticity of the

arteries, i.e. if the arteries are narrowed and inelastic the blood pressure is raised.

4. The rhythm of the heart and the orderly sequence with which the various chambers contract is dependent on specialized neuro-muscular tissue in the heart.

The impulse for each cardiac contraction commences at the sino-atrial node (the pacemaker of the heart) near the entrance of the superior vena cava into the right atrium. It spreads over the muscle of both atria and reaches the atrio-ventricular node, from which it passes down the atrio-ventricular bundle of His. In the inter-ventricular septum, the bundle of His divides into right and left branches and distributes the impulse to contract to the right and left ventricles respectively.

The bundle of His can only pass a certain number of impulses per minute, that is to say, a definite period must elapse after one impulse has passed before the bundle is able to transmit the next. This period of rest during which no impulse can pass is called the refractory period.

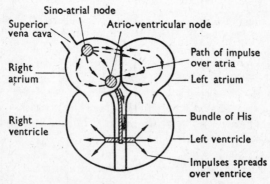

Fig. 4.—Illustrating the spread of the impulse for contraction from the sino-atrial node over the atria to reach the atrio-ventricular node, whence it passes down the bundle of His and is distributed to the ventricles.

5. The constant rate of the heart is maintained because the sino-atrial node is under the influence of two sets of nervous impulses which normally are equally balanced.

Para-sympathetic nerve fibres reaching the heart in the vagus (Xth cranial) nerve carry impulses which tend to slow its rate (inhibitors).

Sympathetic fibres from the cardiac plexus tend to increase its rate (accelerators).

Therefore, drugs which tend to paralyse or depress the para-sympathetic or vagus will permit over-action of the sympathetic and the rate of the heart will be increased. Those which stimulate the vagus (para-sympathetic) will slow the rate.

Conversely, stimulation of the sympathetic fibres will also increase the heart-rate, while their depression will slow the rate by permitting over-action of the vagus.

As an example, adrenaline, which stimulates the sympathetic, will increase the rate of the heart if given by injection or if its secretion by the suprarenal glands is naturally increased as it is in states of fear or violent emotion.

DRUGS ACTING ON THE HEART

The most important drugs acting on the heart itself are those of the digitalis group, and the condition on which they have the most beneficial and dramatic effect is atrial (auricular) fibrillation.

In atrial fibrillation, the atrial muscle loses its power of contracting as a whole, and instead of one impulse commencing at the sino-atrial node spreading in an orderly fashion over the atrial muscle to reach the atrio-ventricular node at the rate of approximately 72 per minute, a series of irregular contractions occur which are scattered over the atria. Each of these small contractions produces an impulse which passes to the atrio-ventricular node. In atrial fibrillation, therefore, this node is bombarded with impulses at the rate of about 400 per minute.

Owing to the refractory period, however, the bundle of His can only transmit a certain number of these irregular impulses. The ventricle therefore contracts at irregular intervals at a rapid rate (often up to 130 beats per minute).

Since the contractions of the ventricle occur at irregular and rapid intervals, it follows that it can never be filled completely nor will it contain the same amount of blood for each beat. Therefore the output per beat is small and variable in quantity. This means that the pulse will also be irregular both in rhythm and volume. Some of the heart beats will be so small that the pulse-wave produced will be imperceptible at the wrist. Therefore the rate of the pulse counted at the wrist will not be a true indication of the rate of the ventricles. Hence the importance of taking and recording both the pulse-rate and the rate at the apex in cases of atrial fibrillation.

The digitalis group

Drugs of the digitalis group act: (i) on the bundle of His in atrial fibrillation. Their action is a depressing one, that is, they lower its power of conducting impulses. In other words, they increase the refractory period. By this means, the bundle of His allows fewer of the irregular impulses bombarding the atrio-ventricular node to pass and, by adjusting the dose of the drug, this number can be reduced to 70 or 80 per minute or even lower.

In this way the ventricular rate is slowed. Slowing of the ventricle means better filling of the ventricle and an increased output per beat. Consequently, the efficiency of the heart as a pump is increased and the general circulation is improved. (ii) Digitalis acts directly on the myocardium and increases the force of systolic contraction. It thereby increases cardiac output and reduces venous congestion and the raised venous pressure in congestive heart failure. This is its most important action.

The improvement in the circulation has other beneficial effects:

1. The circulation in the coronary arteries is increased and the nutrition of the heart is improved.

2. The circulation in the kidneys is improved and the output of urine is increased, a factor important in the reduction of cardiac oedema. This explains the diuretic action of digitalis in heart disease.

3. Oedema is also diminished, by reason of the improved circulation in the more distant and dependent parts of the body.

Summary

The action of the digitalis group of drugs may be summarized:

(i) Digitalis is of special value in atrial (auricular) fibrillation.

(ii) It acts by depressing the bundle of His and increasing its refractory period.

(iii) Thereby it slows ventricular rate, increases the output per beat and improves the circulation.

(iv) Digitalis also has a general tonic effect on the heart muscle, increasing the force of ventricular contraction and the cardiac output. It is, therefore, of value in other cases of cardiac weakness. Its most dramatic effect, however, is in atrial fibrillation.

(v) Improvement in the circulation has a beneficial effect on various symptoms, e.g. the urinary output is increased; oedema is diminished.

(vi) It has an action on the vagus nerve and sino-atrial node which also contributes to the slowing of the cardiac rate.

(vii) In therapeutic doses digitalis has little action on the normal heart.

Digitalis

Digitalis is obtained from the foxglove (*Digitalis purpurea*) and was first used in the treatment of heart disease by Withering in 1785. Many preparations exist, from the simple powdered leaves to pure substances (glycosides) such as digoxin, digitoxin, lanatoside C and Nativelle's 'Digitaline'.

The following are the most important:

Digoxin tablets ('Lanoxin'), 0·25 to 1·0 milligram.

Digoxin injection, BP, for intravenous or intramuscular use, 2 to 4 ml.

Digitalis tablets, BP (sometimes called *Digitalis folia*) 30–100 mg ($\frac{1}{2}$ to $1\frac{1}{2}$ grains).

Nativelle's 'Digitaline' and digitoxin, 0·1–1 mg.

N.B.—60 mg. of digitalis leaves and 0·1 mg of Nativelle's 'Digitaline' are both approximately equivalent in therapeutic effect to 0·25 mg of digoxin.

Methods of administration of digitalis

Treatment of atrial (auricular) fibrillation with digitalis may be divided into stages:

(i) Initial doses or reduction of heart rate to about 70.

(ii) Maintenance doses.

(iii) Urgent cases.

Initial doses. Provided no digitalis has been taken within two or three days, a full dose of digoxin or digitalis tablets is given.

Maintenance doses. These are adjusted to maintain the pulse and apex rate between 60 and 80 per minute. One rest day in seven during which the drug is omitted is often of value.

Urgent cases. In very urgent cases the most rapid results are obtained by giving digoxin; e.g. 1 milligram by mouth will slow the heart rate in 6 to 8 hours. If necessary, 0·75 to 1·0 mg may be given intravenously in 10 to 20 ml. of normal saline. The heart rate begins to fall in 10 minutes and the maximum effect of the dose is apparent in less than 2 hours. Digoxin should not be given by subcutaneous injection.

Notes on the administration of digitalis

1. It was formerly the practice to give digitalis in a mixture containing the tincture. This is most undesirable because unless the mixture is quite fresh, the potency of the tincture is partially destroyed by the water present and, if more than a few days old, it is unreliable in its results.

2. During the treatment of atrial fibrillation with digitalis both the apex rate and the pulse rate should be recorded.

3. The urinary output should be carefully measured.

4. Digitalis is not rapidly absorbed from the alimentary tract, the average dose requiring about 6 hours. There is, therefore, no advantage in giving the drug orally more often than six hourly.

5. The excretion of the drug is also slow and cumulative effects may be seen, hence the value of omitting the drug one day a week. Elderly patients usually require a reduced dosage, because toxic effects occur more readily in old age.

Toxic symptoms

These may be due to over-dosage, cumulative effect or idiosyncrasy. They include:

(i) Undue slowness of the pulse and apex beat, e.g. below 60.

(ii) Coupling of beats (*pulsus bigeminus*) and other cardiac irregularities.

(iii) Nausea and vomiting. Anorexia and diarrhoea may occur.

(iv) Diminished urinary output.

(v) Alterations in the electrocardiogram.

Other drugs of the digitalis group

These are very much less frequently employed than digitalis and are only useful when patients show intolerance to the latter drug. They include strophanthus, ouabain and lanatoside.

Quinidine sulphate [(60–300 mg) 1 to 5 grains]

This is a drug allied to quinine in composition. It acts directly on the heart muscle and, in some cases, by reducing its conductive power is able to restore atrial fibrillation to normal rhythm. Direct current electric shock therapy is now used in preference to this rather dangerous drug.

Quinidine is not suitable for use in all cases of atrial fibrillation and very careful selection is necessary. There are certain dangers in its use, including embolism and toxic symptoms such as diarrhoea, vomiting, skin rashes, convulsions and sudden death.

Technique of administration. A preliminary period of rest in bed with a course of digitalis therapy is generally advisable.

1st day: a test dose of 180 mg (3 grains) is given.

2nd day (if no toxic symptoms are shown by the test dose): 360 mg (6 grains) every 3 hours for 4 doses (total, 1·5 grams, 24 grains).

3rd day: 360 mg (6 grains) every 3 hours for 5 doses (total, 2·0 grams, 30 grains).

4th to 7th days: This dosage is continued. If the drug is successful normal rhythm will be established within this period and may be maintained by a dose of 300 mg (5 grains) once or twice a day.

Its main value is in the condition known as paroxysmal tachycardia, when small doses are given once or twice daily with a view to preventing the recurrence of the condition.

Procainamide ('Pronestyl') (0·5 to 1 gram)

This is a synthetic substance having somewhat similar actions and uses to quinidine in paroxysmal tachycardia. It may be given orally or by very slow intravenous injection (up to 10 ml., and not exceeding 50 mg per minute), during which a check on the blood pressure and electrocardiogram is maintained.

Lignocaine ('Xylocaine') has a similar action but is less likely to cause hypotension. It is given intravenously to reduce or abolish ventricular ectopic beats resulting from myocardial infarction. An initial single dose of 100 mg is usually followed by an infusion of 1–2 mg per minute for up to 48 hr.

Beta-adrenergic-receptor blockade

The sympathetic nervous system excites the heart via what are known as beta receptors. These receptors can be blocked by certain drugs, e.g. propranolol ('Inderal'). This is used in some cases of atrial fibrillation which have failed to respond to digitalis. It is also useful in the treatment of arrhythmias induced by digitalis, some cases of angina pectoris and some cases of hypertension.

Other drugs occasionally used in the treatment of cardiac arrhythmias include methacholine, neostigmine, antalozine and phenytoin.

CIRCULATORY STIMULANTS

Circulatory stimulants are drugs which are given to improve the circulation. They are generally employed in acute conditions such as shock.

D

They may be roughly classified into two main groups:

(i) Those which raise the blood pressure by their action on the arteries (vaso-constrictors).

(ii) Those which stimulate the heart directly.

(a) **Adrenaline** and noradrenaline are examples of drugs which stimulate the alpha-receptors in the walls of small arteries. They cause constriction of the arteries by stimulating the plain muscle in their walls to contract. The result of this general arterial constriction is a rise in blood pressure.

Noradrenaline ('Levophed') is usually given in a slow intravenous drip, 4 ml. of a 1 in 1000 solution being added to 1 litre of saline or 5% dextrose solution (p. 165). Its main use is when the blood pressure is low in surgical shock.

Mephentermine ('Mephine') is used to raise blood pressure in cases of shock and severe collapse, not caused by haemorrhage (e.g. coronary thrombosis). It may be given by intravenous or intramuscular injection in doses of up to 30 mg at intervals until the systolic blood pressure is maintained at 100 mm Hg.

Metaraminol ('Aramine'), 0.5 to 5 mg intravenously, 2 to 10 mg intramuscularly, is a vaso-constrictor used in hypotension due to cardiac infarction, shock or haemorrhage. It is contraindicated in other cases of heart disease, diabetes and thyrotoxicosis.

(b) Certain drugs stimulate the sympathetic beta-receptors of the heart and cause an increase in the rate and force of contraction of this organ. Adrenaline, isoprenaline and orciprenaline are such substances. A long-acting preparation of isoprenaline, 'Saventrine' is particularly useful in the treatment of complete heart block. In patients who fail to respond or in whom adverse effects occur, an electronic pacemaker is usually necessary.

Digitalis is a drug which stimulates the heart to contract more forcibly but does not increase the heart rate. It is therefore said to have an *inotropic* action. In cases in which it also slows the heart, it is said to have a negative *chronotropic* action.

Certain respiratory stimulants (analeptics) were once used as cardiac stimulants. They were only effective, however, when they improved myocardial oxygenation as a secondary effect of stimulating respiration. In other words, they are only of value when ventilation of the lungs is inadequate. Nikethamide ('Coramine'), 2–4 ml. parenterally, is the most popular analeptic.

DRUGS ACTING ON THE ARTERIES

The drugs in this group, which lower blood pressure by dilating the arteries, are called vasodilators. Advantage is taken of both these effects for different conditions, i.e.

(i) Drugs are sometimes used especially for their power of dilating the coronary arteries.

(ii) They may be employed with the definite intention of lowering blood pressure.

(iii) They may be used for their action in dilating the peripheral arteries in the limbs.

DRUGS USED TO DILATE THE CORONARY ARTERIES

The nitrites and nitrates

These drugs are used especially in the treatment of angina pectoris, both in acute attacks and with a view to reducing their frequency. Their main action is to dilate the coronary arteries.

Glyceryl trinitrate tablets (0·5 to 1 mg)

This is the most important drug used in the treatment of angina pectoris, the pain of which is rapidly relieved. It is of greatest value when taken before an exertion which the patient knows, by experience, would usually cause pain. The tablets (*Tabellae glycerylis trinitratis*) are placed under the tongue or chewed very slowly but not swallowed whole. The drug is absorbed by the mucous membrane of the mouth, but has little effect if it enters the stomach.

Its action is more prolonged than that of amyl nitrite (i.e. up to 15 minutes). Kept in a well closed container, in a dark, dry, cool place, tablets can be expected to remain potent for 2 years from the date of their manufacture. In less favourable conditions they may lose their potency in a few months.

Amyl nitrite capsules

This is a volatile liquid given by inhalation. It is supplied in glass capsules containing 0·2 ml. (3 minims), which are broken in a handkerchief and then inhaled. Its action in angina pectoris is rapid but brief. It also dilates the other arteries of the body, and this can be observed in the flushing of the face and felt in the throbbing of the head after inhalation. It is sometimes used to relieve biliary and renal colic and hiccough. Octyl nitrite has a similar action.

'Peritrate' (erythrityl tetranitrate) 20 to 40 mg ($\frac{1}{4}$ to 1 grain), 'Mycardol' (pentaerythritol tetranitrate and 'Vascardin' (sorbide nitrate) are long-acting nitrate preparations taken three or four times a day in the hope of preventing anginal pains. They are contraindicated in glaucoma.

DRUGS USED TO LOWER BLOOD PRESSURE
(hypotensive drugs)

High blood pressure or hypertension is very common, especially with advancing years, and in certain cases it is considered necessary to take steps to lower it.

At one time the operation of sympathectomy was carried out; more recently a number of drugs have been employed although none is always entirely satisfactory.

Some of these drugs act on the sympathetic and parasympathetic nerve ganglia and are referred to as **ganglion blocking agents.** The main effect of this action is to cause dilation of the arterioles, thereby reducing peripheral resistance and, consequently, a lowering of the blood pressure.

Other nerve impulses transmitted through the ganglia may also be affected so that side-effects may occur. These include dry mouth, constipation and possibly paralytic ileus which is very dangerous. Impairment of visual accommodation, difficulty in micturition and even impotence may be noticed.

If the blood pressure is lowered too much, giddiness or faintness on assuming the erect posture may occur (postural hypotension). Over-dosage may produce a severe fall in blood pressure which is treated cautiously with injections of metaraminol.

Examples of ganglion-blocking drugs are:

Hexamethonium	('Vegolysen')
Pentolinium	('Ansolysen')
Mecamylamine	('Iversine')
Pempidine	('Perolysen')

The first two drugs are used parenterally in the treatment of hypertensive emergencies, i.e. hypertensive encephalopathy and acute left ventricular failure. Otherwise, ganglion-blockers are not often used now.

Adrenergic-blocking agents selectively depress the sympathetic nerve fibres and do not affect the parasympathetic nerves. Unpleasant effects of parasympathetic blockade are thus avoided.

Side-effects are common, however. Of these, postural hypotension, diarrhoea and tiredness may be particularly troublesome. **Bretylium** ('Darenthin') was the first of these drugs but tolerance develops readily, so that patients cease to respond. Other adrenergic-blockers are:

Guanethidine ('Ismelin')   **Bethanidine** ('Esbatal')
Guanoxan   ('Envacar')   **Debrisoquine** ('Declinax')

Guanoxan probably lowers blood pressure by central as well as peripheral actions.

Guanethidine is an established and generally satisfactory hypo-tensive agent. It is well absorbed and has a long action. Only one dose daily is required. Treatment is commenced with a dose of 10 mg. Dosage is gradually increased until control is achieved, usually with less than 100 mg daily.

Other drugs

Oral diuretics such as the thiazides and chlorthalidone may, by themselves, control mild hypertension. Their action may be a direct one upon the blood vessels. Potassium supplements are required just as they are when these drugs are used as diuretics.

Rauwolfia compounds. These have a relatively mild hypotensive effect. They also have a sedative effect. **Reserpine** ('Serpasil') is an alkaloid obtained from the roots of Rauwolfia serpentina. Its hypo-tensive action is probably due to depletion of tissue stores of noradrenaline. The most serious side-effect is mental depression, which may lead to suicide. For this reason, rauwolfia compounds are used in small dosage, e.g. 0·5 mg of reserpine daily. This, by itself, is inadequate for the control of hypertension and it is usual to prescribe these drugs together with a diuretic or other hypo-tensive agent. Intramuscular reserpine is sometimes used in hypertensive emergencies.

Methyldopa ('Aldomet') interferes with the synthesis of nor-adrenaline. It is well absorbed when given by mouth and the dose is 0·5 to 4 G daily. Postural hypotension is not usually a problem with this drug because it lowers the supine as well as the standing blood pressure. It is suitable for mild or moderate cases.

Propranolol ('Inderal'), a beta-receptor blocking agent (see p. 16), may be used for the treatment of mild to moderate hyperten-sion unless there are contra-indications such as heart failure or bronchial asthma. It is particularly suitable for the young person with labile hypertension and a high cardiac output. It probably

TABLE 2.—COMMON HYPOTENSIVE DRUGS

Type of drug	Official name	Other names
Ganglion blocking	Hexamethonium	'Vegolysen'
	Mecamylamine	'Minversine'
Adrenergic blocking	Guanethidine	'Ismelin'
	Bethanidine	'Estabal'
	Guanoxan	'Envacar'
	Debrisoquine	'Declinax'
Methyldopa	Methyldopa	'Aldomet'
Rauwolfia alkaloid	Reserpine	'Serpasil'
Diuretics	Chlorothiazide	'Saluric'
	Chlorthalidone	'Hygroton'

acts principally by reducing the cardiac output. The initial dose is 20 mg four times a day and the maintenance dose commonly lies between 60 and 80 mg four times a day.

Clonidine ('Catapres') has both central and peripheral sites of action.

Hydrallazine ('Apresoline') and 'Veriloid' are rarely used.

In the treatment of patients with hypertension any one of these drugs may be used alone or may be given in combination with one of the others, thereby reducing the necessary dose of each substance. In obese patients a reducing diet may also be ordered.

It is important to remember that diuretics such as **chlorothiazide** ('Saluric') and chlorthalidone ('Hygroton') increase considerably the effect of hypotensive drugs, the dose of which may have to be halved when they are given together.

DRUGS USED FOR THEIR ACTION ON THE PERIPHERAL ARTERIES

(i) Alpha-adrenergic-receptor blockade

Certain drugs block the alpha-adrenergic receptors in the walls of the arterioles and so reduce or abolish the vasoconstrictor effect of the sympathetic nervous system. Vasodilatation results. Alpha-adrenergic-blocking agents increase the flow of blood in the skin rather than in muscles, however, and are therefore of use in cases of Raynaud's phenomenon, chilblains and superficial ulcers rather than in cases of intermittent claudication.

Phentolamine ('Rogitine') is a short-acting alpha-adrenergic blocker and is used mainly in the diagnosis of phaeochromocytoma, a tumour of the adrenal medulla which secretes excessive quantities of adrenaline and noradrenaline and thereby causes hypertension.

Phenoxybenzamine ('Dibenyline') is a powerful and long-acting alpha-adrenergic blocker but is not often used because side-effects are common.

Thymoxamine ('Opilon') may be given by direct injection into veins or arteries or may be given orally as a 40 mg tablet, one, four times a day.

(ii) Drugs acting directly on the vessel wall to produce vasodilatation

These include ethyl alcohol, nicotinic acid, inositol nicotinate ('Hexopal'), papaverine and bamethan ('Vasculit').

Tolazoline ('Priscol') has both an alpha-adrenergic-blocking effect and a direct vasodilator effect on peripheral vessels but, even so, blood flow is increased more in skin than in muscles. The oral dose is one or two 25 mg tablets four times a day.

None of these drugs is very effective in intermittent claudication. Progressive walking exercise may produce improvement by increasing the collateral circulation. Some patients, in whom the obliterative changes are mainly in the larger arteries, benefit from arterial surgery—disobliteration or grafting procedures.

Antihistamine drugs

Histamine is a substance which is liberated in the tissues especially in allergic conditions such as hay fever and urticaria and which has an action on the local circulation directly opposite to that of adrenaline. It has a powerful action in dilating capillaries, and may increase their permeability so that plasma escapes into the tissues producing local oedema such as is seen in urticaria.

There are a number of drugs which block the action of histamine known as the antihistamines. They include:

'Thephorin'	(Phenindamine)	25 to 50 mg
'Phenergan'	(Promethazine)	25 to 75 mg
'Benadryl'	(Diphenhydramine)	50 mg
'Histantin'	(Chlorcyclizine)	50 to 100 mg
'Antistin'	(Antazoline)	100 mg
'Anthisan'	(Mepyramine)	100 mg
'Piriton'	(Chlorpheniramine)	4 mg

They are given once, twice or three times a day according to their duration of action and should be taken after meals. They sometimes produce marked drowsiness and should not be taken before driving a car or undertaking work requiring special skill unless their precise effect on the individual is known.

In addition to their value in most allergic conditions, these drugs are also useful in paralysis agitans, travel sickness and for the itching of obstructive jaundice. They are also used in the form of ointments to relieve irritation in some skin conditions and insect bites but may themselves cause dermatitis in sensitive patients.

In severe anaphylactic shock an intravenous preparation may be used following an intravenous injection of hydrocortisone hemi-succinate and a subcutaneous injection of adrenaline.

CHAPTER 8

Drugs Acting on the Blood

Blood consists of red corpuscles, white cells and blood platelets floating in plasma.

THE RED CELLS (ERYTHROCYTES)

The **red corpuscles** or erythrocytes, which number 5,000,000 per cubic millimetre, are biconcave discs containing haemoglobin. Haemoglobin consists of a protein globin, combined with an iron-containing pitment. The red corpuscles are developed in the bone marrow from large nucleated cells called proerythroblasts (pronormoblasts), which as they mature become smaller in size and are called normoblasts. Normoblasts become filled with haemoglobin, lose their nuclei and are then discharged as the fully developed erythrocytes into the general circulation.

In order that the proerythroblast may develop into the normoblast, a special blood-forming or erythrocyte maturing factor is necessary. This is produced by the interaction of the intrinsic factor (of Castle) in the gastric juice with an extrinsic factor in the diet (liver, meat and eggs) which is now known to be vitamin B_{12} and which is stored in the liver. The two factors work together, as originally suggested by Castle, and, in this way, the intrinsic factor aids the absorption of the extrinsic factor (vitamin B_{12}) from the terminal ileum. Folic acid is also necessarv for red-cell synthesis. It is present in green vegetables, liver, kidney and yeast, and is absorbed in the jejunum.

In order that sufficient haemoglobin may be manufactured in the body to fill the normoblast and permit its development into the fully formed red corpuscle, there must be an adequate supply of iron. This is normally taken in the diet especially in liver, meat, eggs, oatmeal, peas, beans and wholemeal bread. It is absorbed mainly in the duodenum and upper jejunum.

In disease, the red corpuscles may either be defective (anaemia) or excessive in number (polycythaemia). Anaemia may be defined as a deficiency in the number of red corpuscles or in the amount of haemoglobin, or both.

Anaemia may be due to:
  Defective blood formation.
  Excessive blood loss.
  Excessive blood destruction.

DRUGS USED FOR DEFECTIVE BLOOD FORMATION

Anaemia due to defective red-cell maturation (megaloblastic anaemia)

Deficiency of vitamin B_{12} or folic acid results in a macrocytic anaemia with a megaloblastic marrow. Dietary deficiency of both vitamins is responsible for cases of tropical macrocytic anaemia. In the U.K. dietary deficiency is rare but folic acid deficiency may occur in elderly people and vitamin B_{12} deficiency may occur in strict vegetarians and in elderly people. Other causes of deficiency are as listed below:

Vitamin B_{12} deficiency
  1. Pernicious (Addisonian) anaemia, in which there is absence of intrinsic factor and hence no absorption of the vitamin B_{12}.
  2. Total (or, sometimes, partial) gastrectomy.
  3. Malabsorption states, e.g. Crohn's disease.
  4. Infestation with the fish tapeworm as the result of eating raw fish, as in Japan.

Folic acid deficiency
  1. Malabsorption states, e.g. tropical sprue.
  2. Macrocytic anaemia of pregnancy.
  3. Haemolytic anaemias and leukaemia.
  4. Folic acid antagonists, e.g. methotrexate, which is used against leukaemia, and phenytoin, primidone and barbiturates which are used as anticonvulsants.
  5. Alcoholic cirrhosis of the liver. In these cases, folic acid deficiency is due to an inadequate diet.

Vitamin B_{12} and liver extracts

Fresh liver is now never used and vitamin B_{12} has replaced liver extracts.

Vitamin B_{12} may be given: (i) by intramuscular injection, which is the usual, more efficient and economical method or (ii) by mouth, which is much less reliable. Different preparations are available for each form of therapy. Treatment is divided into two stages:

1. The therapeutic stage, when large doses are employed until the blood count has reached normal. Injections are given daily or two or three times a week.

2. The maintenance stage, which is continued indefinitely by injections every three or four weeks.

Vitamin B_{12} (**Cyanocobalamin,** 'Cytamen') is usually given by intramuscular injection in doses of 100 to 1000 micrograms. Hydroxocobalamin ('Neo-cytamin') appears to be effective in smaller doses given at longer intervals. For oral administration 'Bioparforte' tablets may be used. None of these preparations has any value as a "tonic".

Folic acid. This is one of the factors in the vitamin B complex which, although it will restore the blood picture in pernicious anaemia to normal will not prevent the development of neurological complications. It should not, therefore be used in this condition.

It is, however, valuable in the treatment of macrocytic anaemia in malabsorption states, pregnancy and malnutrition. Dose: 5–20 mg daily. It is usually given by mouth.

Defective haemoglobin formation

Defective formation of haemoglobin is due to lack of iron. This may result from a deficiency of iron in the diet or defective absorption of iron from the alimentary tract. It may also occur after loss of blood by haemorrhage, when haemoglobin is lost from the body in the red corpuscles and an additional quantity of iron is required for the manufacture of new supplies. Because of foetal requirements iron should be given during pregnancy.

1. **Iron** is given by mouth three times daily, e.g.

Ferrous sulphate (*Tab. ferri sulphatis co.*, NF, 'Fersolate'), 200 mg (3 grains).

Ferrous gluconate, 300 mg (5 grains).

Ferric ammonium citrate (*Ferri et ammonii citras*), 2·4 grams (20 to 40 grains). This can be given in mixture form. It tends to blacken the teeth but may be useful for patients who cannot swallow tablets.

Ferrous carbonate or Blaud's pill or tablet (*Pilula ferri carbonatis*), 2 grams (5 to 30 grains).

N.B.—These daily doses should not be exceeded. Special proprietary preparations have little advantage.

2. Various preparations of iron may be given by careful intravenous injections. They are rarely necessary and only indicated when iron absorption is shown to be defective or the patient cannot be trusted to take tablets.

e.g. Saccharated iron oxide ('Ferrivenin').

These are specially prepared solutions which may cause soreness of the arm or phlebitis if they escape from the vein. Occasionally serious collapse may follow an injection. After an initial dose of 2·5 ml., 5 ml. (containing 100 mg), or 10 ml. doses may be given daily or on alternate days until the required amount of iron has been administered, according to the formula

$$\frac{100 - \text{estimated haemoglobin}}{100} \times 2500 \text{ mg}$$

3. 'Imferon' is an iron dextran–complex which may be given by intramuscular injection. The usual dose is 5 ml. When given by intramuscular injection, great care must be taken to see that none of the solution remains in the needle track. Otherwise some permanent staining of the skin may result. 'Jectofer', an iron–sorbitol–citric acid complex, is another intramuscular iron preparation.

Iron poisoning

There is a danger that young children may mistake iron tablets for sweets which will result in severe toxic or even fatal symptoms. The treatment of acute iron poisoning is to administer 'Desferal' intravenously, (25 mg per kg. body weight) in saline. The drug can also be given by mouth.

Excessive blood loss

In severe haemorrhage there is loss of red corpuscles, haemoglobin and fluid (plasma), and the ideal treatment is their replacement by blood transfusion. The loss of fluid, which is even more important than the loss of haemoglobin, can also be made up by giving water by mouth, or saline by rectal, subcutaneous, intravenous and intraperitoneal infusions. Injections of Dextran and plasma transfusions are also of value.

Residual anaemia due to deficiency of haemoglobin requires treatment with iron. Liver extract and vitamin B_{12} are of no value in anaemia of this type because there is no deficiency of anti-anaemic factor.

Excessive blood destruction

There are many causes of haemolytic anaemia, in which the red cells are broken up (lysed). In haemolytic disease of the newborn, treatment consists of exchange transfusion of blood. In other haemolytic anaemias, steroids (e.g. prednisone) may be prescribed or splenectomy may be advised.

Excessive blood formation

In a disease known as polycythaemia (Osler's disease) in which the spleen is enlarged, and also in certain other circumstances, the number of red corpuscles may be considerably increased above the normal (up to 8 or 10 million per c.mm.). Symptoms are relieved by venesection, which is repeated as often as necessary. Radioactive phosphorus (^{32}P) is the most effective treatment for this condition.

THE WHITE CELLS (LEUCOCYTES)

There are two important varieties of white cell, the polymorphonuclear leucocyte, having a granular cytoplasm (granulocyte), and the lymphocyte. The former develop in the bone marrow, the latter in the lymphoid tissue (e.g. the lymph glands and spleen). The normal number of white cells in the blood is 4000 to 10,000 per cubic millimetre, of which about 70 per cent are polymorphonuclear leucocytes and 30 per cent lymphocytes. If the total number of white cells is less than 4000 per c.mm the condition is known as leucopoenia, if more than 10,000 per c.mm it is called leucocytosis.

Acute leukaemias

Leukaemia is a disease in which very large numbers of abnormal white cells (e.g. up to 100,000 or more) are present in the blood.

Drugs used to induce remission

Two drugs are often used in combination.

Steroids, e.g. prednisone 40 mg daily.

Vincristine ('Oncovin'), 2 mg per square metre of body surface area, given intravenously. The dose is repeated after one week.

Rubidomycin, 1 mg/kg of body weight intravenously daily for 1–5 days.

Cytosine arabinoside, 2–3 mg/kg of body weight intravenously daily.

Thioguanine, 2·5 mg/kg of body weight daily by mouth.

Colaspase (L-aspariginase, 'Crasnitin'.)

Maintenance therapy

Drugs are usually used in the following order:

6-mercaptopurine ('Puri-nethol') 2·5 mg/kg of body weight daily by mouth.

Methotrexate ('Amethopterin') 20 mg/sq. metre of body surface area orally or intramuscularly at intervals of 4 days.

Cyclophosphamide ('Endoxana'), 3 mg/kg of body weight daily by mouth.

Chronic myeloid leukaemia

Any of the following drugs may be used, but busulphan is usually tried first.

Busulphan ('Myleran'), 0·065 mg/kg of body weight daily by mouth.

Radioactive phosphorus, ^{32}P.

Dibromomannitol, 750 mg daily, in divided doses, for 4–6 days.

Hydroxyurea ('Hydrea'), 80 mg/kg of body weight twice weekly by mouth.

Mitobronitol ('Myelobromol'), 250 mg daily initially.

Chronic lymphatic leukaemia

Chlorambucil ('Leukeran'), 0·15 mg/kg of body weight daily by mouth or Cyclophosphamide ('Endoxana').

Prednisone as a temporary measure.

The nurse is not expected to commit these doses to memory; they are given merely for reference. There are, in any case, several alternative dosage schemes for the treatment of each of the various types of leukaemia.

DRUGS PRODUCING LEUCOPOENIA

In addition to their reduction in diseases such as typhoid fever, the white cells, especially the polymorphonuclear leucocytes, may be seriously diminished (granulocytopoenia) or completely absent (agranulocytosis) as a result of the toxic action of certain drugs. These drugs are given for other purposes, but it is important to remember this dangerous effect in persons who show idiosyncrasy to them.

The most important drugs liable to produce severe leucopoenia (granulocytopoenia or agranulocytosis) are:

Thiouracil and its derivatives.	Chloramphenicol.
	Troxidone.
The sulphonamides.	Methoin.
Amidopyrine.	Phenylbutazone ('Butazolidin').
Gold salts.	Radioactive substances.

DRUGS PRODUCING THROMBOCYTOPOENIA

Some drugs may interfere with the production of platelets, which results in purpura:

e.g. Phenylbutazone.	Quinidine.
Chlorpropamide.	'Sedormid'.
Tolbutamide.	Sulphonamides.

THE VOLUME OF THE BLOOD

The total volume of the blood is made up by the plasma and the blood cells. It may be decreased by loss of both in severe haemorrhage. The fluid portion alone may be diminished in states of dehydration due to excessive fluid loss from the tissues in severe vomiting, diarrhoea, diabetic coma, severe burns and insufficient fluid intake, i.e. the plasma becomes more concentrated.

The treatment of these conditions necessitates the replacement of fluid by one of the following means:

(i) Blood transfusion, indicated when both plasma and red corpuscles have been lost by haemorrhage.

(ii) Plasma transfusion, especially in cases of shock but also of value after haemorrhage.

(iii) Dextran by intravenous injection.

(iv) Normal saline by rectal, subcutaneous, intravenous or intraperitoneal injection in any case of fluid loss.

(v) Normal saline with glucose by rectal or intravenous injection.

(vi) Water or half-strength normal saline by mouth.

Blood transfusion

The main indications are:

1. Severe haemorrhage

(*a*) Accidents.

(*b*) Before and after operation.

(*c*) Conditions such as haematemesis, abortion, and post-partum haemorrhage.

2. Medical conditions

(*a*) Severe hypochromic anaemia.

(*b*) Some cases of septicaemia.

(*c*) Haemophilia.

(*d*) Occasionally in pernicious anaemia.

It has been found that, for purposes of blood transfusion, individuals may be divided into four groups, and it is only when they belong to the same group that their bloods will mix properly. If blood from the wrong group is transfused the red cells in it are destroyed with very serious and often fatal results to the recipient. It is, therefore, most important to discover the group to which the patient belongs and to select a suitable donor. It is also necessary to test the blood for Rhesus factor (Rh).

In view of the danger to life if blood of the wrong group is given, any nurse handling bottles of blood for transfusion must be particularly careful to see that they reach the right patient, as confusion can occur, especially if more than one transfusion is going on at the same time. Before each bottle is given its label and group should be checked by two persons and compared with the known group of the patient.

TABLE 3.—BLOOD GROUPS.

International	AB	A	B	0
Percentage of persons	5	40	10	45

There is an exception to this rule concerning what are called group O donors. In most instances their blood may be given to any patient without causing ill effects, and they are, therefore, referred to as universal donors, but even with these donors a preliminary test must be made to ensure compatibility.

As a rule, 1000 ml or more of blood are given as a single transfusion in units of 500 ml.

The continuous drip method is generally used, and by this means as much as 3 litres (about 5 pints) or more may be given over a period of 24 hours at the rate of about 40 drops a minute.

The basis of modern blood-transfusion technique is to collect blood from a donor into a vacuum bottle containing a special solution of sodium citrate to prevent clotting. Blood thus obtained can be stored in a cold place for about two weeks.

Packed cell transfusion

"Concentrated human red blood corpuscles" is whole human blood from which 40 per cent of the plasma has been removed. This form of transfusion may be used in certain cases of anaemia when it is especially desirable to raise the haemoglobin rapidly without introducing a large amount of fluid into the circulation.

Plasma transfusion

Plasma will keep longer than citrated blood containing red cells and therefore plasma may be withdrawn from citrated blood after the red corpuscles have fallen by sedimentation to the bottom of the collecting bottle, and stored for a long period.

Plasma is of great value in restoring the blood volume in cases of shock. It may be stored in dry form. Dry plasma is rendered suitable for intravenous injection by dissolving 20 grams in 500 ml. of sterile 5% dextrose in distilled water and using it at once.

Human blood serum may also be used in the same way and can be stored in dry form.

Electrolyte and water replacement solutions
(saline solutions etc.)

The blood and tissue fluids normally contain a more or less constant concentration of various salts, and one of the functions of the kidneys is to keep this at a steady level. If the concentration of salts in the blood is increased there will be a passage of fluid from the tissues to the blood until the salt concentration of both is again equal (i.e. a passage from the weaker to the stronger to produce equality).

The effect produced by this concentration of salts (and other substances) is called osmotic pressure, and, in the example just given, the osmotic pressure in the blood would be greater than that in the tissues and, as a result, water would be withdrawn from the latter until the osmotic pressures of the blood and tissue fluids were equal.

Solutions of salts and other substances are frequently injected into the blood streams for various therapeutic purposes, or they may be applied externally to wounds, etc. Depending on their strength (concentration) such solutions may have the same osmotic pressure as the blood, when they are said to be isotonic (iso=equal). Their strength may be less than that of the blood and, if injected, would have a weakening or diluting effect (hypotonic), or they may be stronger solutions (hypertonic). Hypotonic solutions are not often used in therapeutics.

Sodium chloride injection (normal or isotonic saline)

The term saline used in this connection refers to a solution of sodium chloride or common salt, and normal saline is a sterile solution of sodium chloride in water having a strength of 0·9 per cent.

The concentration of sodium chloride being the same as that of the various salts in the blood, when normal saline is injected intravenously it does not affect the balance which exists between the blood and tissue fluids—unless this is already abnormal and the saline is given to restore the balance to normal.

Hypertonic saline

This is a solution of sodium chloride in water exceeding the strength of normal saline (0·9 per cent). Various concentrations are employed according to the purposes for which they are needed.

When given by intravenous injection, the effect will be to raise the salt concentration in the blood so that it is higher than that in the tissues. The result of this is the withdrawal of fluid from the tissues.

For example, 30 ml. of 30% saline (or 50 ml. of 15 per cent) may be injected intravenously in cases of raised intracranial pressure. The effect is withdrawal of fluid from the brain into the blood. In consequence the brain shrinks in size, thus lowering the tension within the cranium. The more usual practice, however, is to inject 50 ml. of 50% sucrose. A similar effect is produced more slowly by the rectal injection of hypertonic magnesium sulphate solutoin (6 ounces of 25 per cent).

Hypertonic saline is also applied as a wound dressing and by its hypertonic action promotes the flow of tissue fluids into the wound.

Sodium chloride and dextrose injection (glucose–saline solution)
This consists of 4·3% glucose and 0·18% sodium chloride.

Being isotonic it may be injected intravenously or intra-muscularly or subcutaneously with hyaluronidase ('Hyalase').

Dextrose injection (5 per cent) may be given intravenously. In addition to water it also supplies calories having food value.

Hypertonic glucose solutions up to 25 per cent are sometimes used for special purposes.

Potassium chloride injection
Potassium supplements may be required in patients on long-term diuretics which increase potassium excretion and in cases of starvation and severe diarrhoea and vomiting. Because it is cardio-toxic and an irritant it must be diluted 50 times with sodium chloride injection before being given intravenously. If dextrose is included it may be given undiluted.

Sodium lactate injection and **sodium bicarbonate injection**. These are sometimes required.

Dextran injection. This must not be confused with dextrose. Dextran in normal saline is sometimes given intravenously in cases of severe haemorrhage when blood is not available for transfusion and also in cases of shock as a temporary measure. It is made up to have the same osmotic pressure as blood. Its main effect is to increase the blood volume and has the advantage over normal saline that is not so rapidly excreted and, therefore, exercises its action for a longer period after injection.

Gum acacia (6 per cent) has been similarly employed.

Hartmann's solution (*Injectio sodii lactatis composita*, BP) may be given orally, subcutaneously or intravenously in the treatment of gastro-enteritis in children and other conditions when acidosis is present. It contains lactic acid and the chlorides of sodium, potassium and calcium.

Hyaluronidase ('Hyalase'). This is an enzyme found in various animal tissues and may be described as a "spreading factor". That is to say, it increases the permeability of the capillaries and tissues so that substances injected into the latter can be more easily dispersed and more rapidly absorbed into the blood stream.

This is of particular value when intravenous therapy is imposs-ible. Hyaluronidase has many uses, in particular the administration of subcutaneous saline (e.g. in infants) and for pyelograms when a vein cannot be used. 1 ml., containing 1000 units in distilled water, is injected into the site of the proposed infusion. The solution must be freshly prepared.

Substances such as potassium citrate which can prevent clotting when added to blood after it has been withdrawn from the body have already been mentioned (p. 56).

The ability of blood to clot is one of Nature's processes which protects the individual against excessive bleeding as a result of injury.

The actual mechanism is a complicated one and involves the interaction of a number of substances present in the blood, the liver and the tissues. It may be briefly simplified in the following way:

$$1. \quad \text{Blood} = \begin{cases} \text{corpuscles} \\ + \\ \text{plasma} = \end{cases} \begin{cases} \text{fibrin} \\ + \\ \text{serum} \end{cases} = \text{clot.}$$

2. (a) Prothrombin + thromboplastin + calcium $\rightarrow$ thrombin.
    (b) Thrombin + fibrinogen $\rightarrow$ clot.

In greater detail:

1. Blood platelets + factors VIII, IX, XI and XII + calcium $\rightarrow$ Thromboplastin.

2. Thromboplastin + factors V, VII and X + calcium $\rightarrow$ Activated Thromboplastin.

3. Prothrombin + activated thromboplastin $\rightarrow$ Thrombin.

4. Thrombin + fibrinogen + factor VIII $\rightarrow$ fibrin clot.

Clotting of blood within the blood vessels, or thrombosis, is not an uncommon pathological condition. There are drugs which can be given internally which prevent or diminish the risk of clotting within the body. These are referred to as anticoagulants and are of two main types:

1. Heparin.

2. The oral anticoagulants ('Dindevan', 'Sinthrome', 'Marevan').

The two groups of drugs act at different stages of the clotting process.

1. Heparin

This is an anticoagulant substance prepared from beef lung. It acts rapidly and is soon eliminated from the system. It is usually given by intravenous injection in doses of 8000 to 10,000 units every six hours. In order to facilitate this a special needle with a non-leaking diaphragm may be left in the vein if desired, or 1500 units per hour may be given in a saline drip, after a starting dose of 5000 units.

Heparin may be given by intramuscular injection, using a very fine needle, but there is risk of local haematoma formation. It is absorbed slowly and its action is less reliable when given by this route. If the administration of heparin is prolonged, the dosage is controlled by estimating the clotting time of the blood.

Overdosage. The antidote to overdosage is the intravenous injection of protamine sulphate, 50 mg of which will neutralize the effect of 5000 units of heparin. A blood transfusion may also be given.

2. Oral anticoagulants

These substances differ from each other somewhat in chemical composition but all act by preventing the formation of prothrombin and other factors (VII, IX and X) in the liver. Thus they take some time to act since the clotting factors present in the blood must first be used up.

Phenindione. ('Dindevan') belongs to the indanedione group of drugs and is given in doses of 100 mg b.d. followed by 50 mg usually twice daily.

Nicoumalone. ('Sinthrome') is supplied in 1 mg and 4 mg tablets. The average dose is: 1st day 8–16 mg, 2nd day 4–12 mg, 3rd and subsequent days 1–6 mg.

Warfarin sodium ('Marevan'). Initial dose 25–50 mg; subsequent doses 3–15 mg daily.

Since these drugs take 24 to 36 hours to become effective, it is a common practice to commence anticoagulant therapy with heparin for twenty-four to thirty-six hours, during which the first tablets of 'Dindevan' or 'Sinthrome' are beginning to act. Their dosage is controlled by estimations of the blood prothrombin time, which should be kept at 2 to $2\frac{1}{2}$ times the control time, or the 'Thrombotest' value which should be kept at $7\frac{1}{2}$ to 15 per cent of the control.

Overdosage may be followed by bleeding into the skin and mucous membrances (purpura), the presence of red cells in the urine (haematuria), vaginal haemorrhage or excessive haemorrhage from recent wounds or operation sites. The treatment is to stop the drug at once and to give blood transfusions and intravenous vitamin K_1,

5 to 20 mg. (Ordinary water-soluble vitamin K is ineffective in this condition.)

Haemorrhagic effects may result not only from overdosage of an anti-coagulant but also from giving certain drugs to patients who are receiving anti-coagulant therapy. These drugs include aspirin, phenylbutazone, chlorpropamide, clofibrate and broad-spectrum antibiotics.

Anticoagulants are used in the treatment of coronary artery thrombosis, pulmonary embolism and thrombosis of veins in the limbs, etc. They do not dissolve clot once it has formed, but prevent either the development of, or extension of, thrombosis.

The human body possesses a chemical mechanism, known as the fibrinolytic system, for lysing (breaking up) fibrin, hence dissolving thrombus. This system can be activated by urokinase or strepto-kinase ('Kabikinase'). Unfortunately the latter, being a product of bacteria, causes the formation of antigens in man, so that a second course of treatment may result in an allergic reaction. Urokinase is difficult to prepare and is not available in large quantities.

CHAPTER 9

Drugs Acting on the Respiratory System

For purposes of therapeutics it is convenient to consider separately the lower respiratory tract, consisting of the trachea, bronchi and alveoli of the lungs; and the upper respiratory tract which includes the nose, pharynx and larynx.

The object of respiration is the interchange of gases between the blood and the atmosphere, oxygen being absorbed and carbon dioxide (and water) being excreted by the lungs.

The rate and depth of respiration is controlled by the respiratory centre in the medulla oblongata in such a way that the concentration of oxygen and carbon dioxide in the blood is normally kept constant. This is done in the following way: The respiratory centre is especially sensitive to the amount of carbon dioxide in the blood. If this rises above the normal (e.g. as a result of exercise) the respiratory centre is stimulated so that the rate and depth of respiration are increased. The increase in the respiratory movements results in a greater intake of oxygen and an increased excretion of carbon dioxide, so that the concentration of the latter in the blood tends to fall to normal once more.

Other substances may also influence the respiratory centre. They may produce similar stimulation, with increased movements, or alternatively they may depress the centre so that breathing becomes slower and shallower.

The respiratory tract is lined with ciliated epithelium, the cells of which also secrete mucus. The bronchioles have plain muscle fibres in their walls.

There are two troublesome features which occur in a number of disorders affecting the respiratory system viz.:

1. Cough.
2. Bronchospasm.

A cough is a reflex act having a cough centre in the medulla. The stimulus provoking a cough may arise from irritation or inflamma-

111

tion in the pharynx, larynx, trachea, bronchi, lungs or pleura. It may be:

(*a*) dry and unproductive; (*b*) loose and with sputum.

(*a*) Sometimes it is desirable to suppress a distressing dry cough by means of a sedative linctus containing drugs which depress the cough reflex by acting on the centre.

(*b*) Expectorant drugs may be needed to loosen sticky sputum.

DRUGS STIMULATING THE RESPIRATORY CENTRE

It has already been seen that cardiac and respiratory stimulants (analeptics) are closely allied and that an increase in respiration has a beneficial effect on the heart by increasing its oxygen supply (p. 90). The stimulants of the respiratory centre are, therefore, used to counteract its depression in various types of poisoning, during anaesthesia and other conditions in which respiratory failure may be evident. They include:

Nikethamide ('Coramine') Caffeine
Aminophylline (p. 118) Ethamivan ('Vandid')
Bemegride ('Megimide') Carbon dioxide
Nalorphine ('Lethidrone')

Nalorphine ('Lethidrone') is used when the depression is due to morphine.

Carbon dioxide

Carbon dioxide (CO_2) is a colourless gas which plays a number of important parts in the economy of Nature. It is an oxide of the element carbon and is produced when carbon is burnt in the presence of sufficient oxygen. It must not be confused with carbon monoxide (CO), a very poisonous oxide of carbon, which is present in large amounts in domestic coal gas.

Carbon dioxide is present in the atmospheric air, i.e. inspired air (0·04 per cent), and in expired air (4 per cent). It is soluble in water. In the manufacture of "soda water", the gas is dissolved in water under pressure. Owing to the escape of carbon dioxide the solution effervesces when the pressure is withdrawn. Beer, champagne and effervescing mineral waters ("aerated waters") also give off carbon dioxide.

It can be compressed by pumping it into steel cylinders and, by special methods, can be converted into a solid, soft, snowlike substance, "carbon dioxide snow", which only remains solid at a very low temperature.

The main use of carbon dioxide is as a respiratory stimulant. Mixtures containing 5 to 10 per cent of carbon dioxide with oxygen are administered by inhalation. The additional concentration of carbon dioxide thus produced in the lungs leads to an increase in the amount in the blood. The respiratory centre is, therefore, stimulated so that respiration is increased in frequency and depth. A mixture of carbon dioxide 5 per cent with oxygen 95 per cent may be administered, using a B.L.B. type of mask, in carbon monoxide poisoning. In a severe case, however, only hyperbaric oxygen therapy may save the patient's life.

It is useful in helping the expansion of the lungs after any portion has been collapsed, e.g. postoperative "atelectasis", and after abdominal operations when the action of the diaphragm may have been impaired.

A solution of carbon dioxide in water, e.g. "soda water", has a mildly stimulating effect on the mucous membrane of the stomach, improving the appetite and causing a feeling of well-being. Effervescing waters are therefore of value in cases of gastric catarrh. The increased blood supply to the mucous membrane caused by this stimulating effect hastens the absorption of water and other substances which accounts for the rapid absorption of alcohol from sparkling wines such as champagne and may explain their exceptionally exhilarating effect.

In solid form, **"carbon dioxide snow"**, which can be produced in the shape of a cone or pencil, is applied to the skin in the treatment of naevi, moles, warts, etc., on which it has a freezing action. If contact is too prolonged blister formation may ensue.

Oxygen

Although not a respiratory stimulant, oxygen may be conveniently considered here on account of its use in cases of respiratory failure.

The atmosphere (inspired air) contains 20 per cent oxygen and the expired air 16 per cent. The 4 per cent oxygen absorbed via the alveoli of the lungs into the blood is conveyed in the red corpuscles to the tissues as oxyhaemoglobin.

The amount of oxygen carried to the tissues may be *decreased* by (*a*) diseases of the lungs and disorders of the pulmonary circulation, whereby the blood fails to acquire sufficient oxygen during its passage through the lungs.

(*b*) General circulatory failure with stagnation of blood in the peripheral parts.

(*c*) Deficiency in the oxygen-carrying power of the blood due to decrease in the amount of haemoglobin or red corpuscles, i.e. anaemia.

(*d*) Defective oxygen-carrying power of haemoglobin by its conversion into carboxyhaemoglobin in gas (carbon monoxide) poisoning.

The amount of oxygen in the blood can only be *increased* by increasing the amount of oxygen in the alveolar air. This may be done by the administration of oxygen by inhalation.

Oxygen may be given in the following ways:

1. The oxygen tent, the ideal method for children.

2. Oxygen mask. Several types are available. Some (e.g. the B.L.B. mask) employ the principle of re-breathing. The Pneumask is a disposable plastic mask of this type. Where there is a risk of carbon dioxide narcosis, rebreathing of expired gas is undesirable. Thus in respiratory failure a non-rebreathing mask is required. The Ventimask, incorporating a Venturi device, is very suitable.

The ideal administration of oxygen by any method requires some sort of flow meter with a fine adjustment valve in order that economical and efficient use may be obtained. The amount of oxygen usually required is 2 to 6 litres per minute.

In many hospitals oxygen is piped to each bedside from a central supply.

(*a*) A 100 cubic foot oxygen cylinder with a rate of flow of 4 litres per minute will last about 12 hours.

(*b*) No oil or lubricant must be put on the high-pressure valves as this may cause fire.

(*c*) Under no circumstances should matches or cigarettes be brought near to a patient having oxygen.

Oxygen given by the tube and funnel method does not raise the oxygen content of the alveolar air sufficiently to have any effect. It therefore has no use other than impressing anxious relatives that something is being done, and is a waste of oxygen.

Passing oxygen through water in a Woulf's bottle at a rate at which bubbles can just be counted supplies less than 0·5 litre per minute. This is insufficient to produce any really beneficial effect.

The greatest care must be taken to discriminate between (*a*) pure oxygen and (*b*) oxygen and carbon dioxide mixtures. The latter should only be used when specially ordered.

Particular care is also necessary not to administer oxygen for too long or in too great a concentration to premature and newborn infants. Blindness due to a condition known as retrolental fibroplasia may be caused by excess.

Hyperbaric oxygen

This is oxygen administered under pressure, usually thrice atmospheric pressure or less. It may be used either in a large chamber of compressed air shared by the patient's attendants or in an individual tank only large enough for the patient. The former chamber is known as a walk-in pressure vessel and the latter is known as a single-patient pressure vessel or hyperbaric bed. In the large chamber, oxygen is administered in the usual manner by a closely-fitting mask or by endotracheal tube; the high atmospheric pressure ensures a high concentration of dissolved oxygen in the tissues. Surgical operations may, if necessary, be performed in the chamber. In the hyperbaric bed, the patient sits or lies alone for short periods (up to 2–3 hours). In this, the oxygen itself is usually the compressing gas and the need for a mask is obviated.

Hyperbaric oxygen is used for the treatment of gas gangrene, carbon monoxide poisoning, the "bends", air embolism and surface infections.

DRUGS WHICH DEPRESS THE RESPIRATORY CENTRE

There are a number of drugs which slow the rate and diminish the depth of respiration. They are not, however, employed therapeutically to produce this result and this action must be regarded as a side effect of their uses for other purposes for example:

All general anaesthetics.
Morphine.
Alcohol.
Barbiturates.
Chloral and other hypnotics in toxic doses.

Cough-suppressants

Drugs which reduce the excitability of the respiratory centre and are thereby effective in diminishing a dry and unproductive cough include:

Morphine and opium	Methadone ('Physeptone')
Diamorphine (Heroin)	Pholcodine ('Ethnine' etc.)
Codeine	

These drugs are often employed in various linctuses which are made up with syrup. The dose is usually 5 ml.

　　Squill opiate linctus (*Linctus scillae opiatus*)
　　Codeine linctus (*Linctus codeinae*)
　　'Physeptone' linctus
　　Pholcodine linctus (*Linctus pholcodine*)

Other linctuses contain noxapine; examples are 'Coscopin' and 'Extil'. There are in fact an enormous number of proprietary cough medicines the respective merits of which are difficult to compare.

Sucking a sweet or medicated lozenge (e.g. liquorice) will often help a troublesome cough.

DRUGS AFFECTING BRONCHIAL SECRETION

Expectorants

An expectorant may be defined as a drug which aids the expulsion of mucus from the respiratory tract either by increasing its secretion or by "loosening" it so that it becomes less tenacious and sticky.

Recent research indicates that many of the drugs which were formerly regarded as increasing the amount of mucus secreted, probably do not act in this way and that they owe their usefulness to their "loosening" effect, which makes expectoration of sputum easier. There is little doubt, however, that in practice the so-called cough mixture is appreciated by the patient and that it relieves his symptoms.

In smaller doses, a number of emetic drugs (p. 62), such as ipecacuanha, act as expectorants. Potassium iodide in addition to other effects, also appears to increase and loosen secretion from the respiratory mucous membrane. It will be remembered that one of the symptoms of "iodism" is that of a common cold in which the flow of mucus from the nose and bronchi is increased (p. 27).

The following are among the important expectorants and one or more are often combined in cough mixtures:

| Ammonium bicarbonate | Potassium iodide |
| Ipecacuanha | Squill |

　　e.g. Ammonia and ipecacuanha mixture (*Misturae ammoniae et ipecacuanhae*), known also as Mistura Expectorans.

Squill (*Scilla*)

In addition to its effect on the heart which, in appropriate doses is similar to that of digitalis, squill also acts as an expectorant by reason of its irritating effect on the bronchial mucous membrane. It is, therefore, more suited to cases of chronic than of acute bronchitis. It is an irritating drug and in large doses acts as a gastro-intestinal irritant and irritant to the kidneys.

Bronchial secretion may be loosened and expectoration helped by the following:

(*a*) Sodium chloride mixture (*Mist. sodii, chlor. co.*) taken in hot water.

(*b*) Steam inhalations to which may be added Benzoin (Friar's balsam) inhalation.

(*c*) Water-mist inhalations, produced by bubbling oxygen through water in a special apparatus. The liquefaction of mucus is increased if ascorbic acid and an oxidizing agent are added to the water. A suitable preparation is 'Ascoxal'.

(*d*) Aerosols containing detergents, e.g. 'Alevaire'.

(*e*) Nebulized 20% solution of acetylcysteine ('Airbron').

(*f*) **Bromhexine** ('Bisolvon') reduces sputum viscosity ("thickness") by disrupting the feltwork of acid mucopolysaccharide (AMPS) fibres which make mucoid sputum viscid. It is therefore used in chronic bronchitis. Dose 8 to 16 mg three times a day.

Anti-expectorants

By this term is meant drugs which reduce bronchial secretion; the most important being belladonna and its alkaloid, atropine. Stramonium has a similar effect. Atropine is used before general anaesthetics, especially ether, in order to prevent excessive bronchial secretion. It is also occasionally given in cases of pulmonary oedema (see also p. 168).

Bronchodilators

These are sometimes referred to as antispasmodics or spasmolytic drugs. They are mainly used in the treatment of bronchial asthma and in some cases of bronchitis, when the plain muscle of the walls of the bronchioles is contracted and in spasm or are oedematous, thus diminishing the airways and causing respiratory distress.

There are two main groups of drugs viz:

1. Sympathomimetic drugs which act on the adrenergic receptor sites in the bronchi.

2. Drugs derived from theophylline which act directly on the bronchial muscle.

Sympathomimetic drugs (see also p. 163)

These include adrenaline, isoprenaline, ephedrine.
They are of relatively short duration of action but this is slightly increased if they are combined with atropine methonitrate.

Adrenaline: subcutaneous injection of 1 in 1000 solution may be given in doses up to 1 ml.

Isoprenaline: this has a similar action to adrenaline and may be given as a 20 mg tablet which is allowed to dissolve under the tongue.

Both these drugs can be used in an aerosol spray for inhalation but patients should be warned of the dangers of overdosage from too frequent use.

Ephedrine may be given by mouth (15 to 60 mg) but may cause insomnia and urinary retention in older subjects. It can, however, be very useful in children.

Salbutamol ('Ventolin') is a beta-adrenergic stimulant. It stimulates those receptors in the bronchi in particular, whereas the other drugs in this group stimulate all beta-receptors, including those in the heart. Salbutamol is, therefore, much less likely to cause undesirable increases in the pulse rate. It may be inhaled from an aerosol or taken in tablet form.

Theophylline

Derivatives of this drug can be very useful. They include: aminophylline, choline theophyllinate ('Choledyl'), and theophylline sodium glycinate ('Englate').

Aminophylline ('Cardophyllin' or Theophylline with Ethylene-diamine)

This drug has a number of actions. It acts on the heart and reduces venous pressure in congestive heart failure. It is also helpful in angina pectoris. Bronchospasm is relieved, hence it is often employed in the treatment of bronchial asthma, especially if there has been no relief from adrenaline or isoprenaline. It is also of value in nocturnal dyspnoea in heart disease ("cardiac asthma") when one or two suppositories may be given at night. Intravenous aminophylline will often abolish Cheyne–Stokes breathing. It also has a mild diuretic action. It may be given by mouth but may cause gastric irritation (up to 500 mg), suppository, or slow intra-venous injection (250 mg in 10 ml.). Intramuscular injection is often painful.

'Choledyl' (choline theophyllinate). This drug has an action similar to aminophylline but is less irritating to the stomach. Dose: 100–400 mg.

Theophylline sodium glycinate ('Englate') available in tablets and as a linctus is useful for mild bronchospasm.

Both 'Choledyl' and 'Englate' are very useful drugs in acute or chronic bronchitis when the chest is wheezy.

Disodium chromoglycate ('Intal') is used in bronchial asthma but is not a bronchodilator. It inhibits allergic reactions in the bronchi and is, therefore, employed prophylactically. It is supplied in capsules ('Spincaps') which contain powder for inhalation via a special insufflator (the 'Spinhaler'). The contents of one 'Spincap' are inhaled every 3 to 6 hours.

Stramonium

In large doses, stramonium has an effect on the nervous system which makes it of value in reducing the muscular rigidity present in Parkinsonism (paralysis agitans). When very large doses are given they have a similar effect to atropine and diminish bronchial secretion and make the mouth dry. To counteract this, pilocarpine, 6 mg ($\frac{1}{10}$ grain), is administered at the same time.

Preparation: Tincture of stramonium (*Tinctura stramonii*), 2 ml. (5 to 30 minims).

In Parkinsonism the dose may be gradually increased to 4 ml. (60 minims) or more.

Lobelia

This may be combined with stramonium in cough mixtures. The important alkaloid lobeline, which stimulates the respiratory centre, is obtained from lobelia.

N.B.—Steroid preparations may be required in status asthma-ticus which fails to respond to other remedies.

Pulmonary antiseptics

Drugs such as creosote and guaiacol which were formerly used as pulmonary antiseptics have now been replaced by sulphona-mides, 'Septrin', penicillin and other antibiotics such as tetracycline which are selected according to the sensitivity of the organisms found in the sputum in bronchitis, pneumonia, lung abscess and bronchiectasis.

DRUGS USED IN RADIOGRAPHY OF THE CHEST

Propyliodone ('Dionosil') and similar preparations (p. 43) are introduced into the trachea from which, by adjusting the position of the patient, they run into the bronchi of either lung. The following methods may be employed: (i) A nasal catheter is passed so that its end over-hangs the larynx and the oil drops down. (ii) The oil is dropped from a special syringe over the back of the tongue. (iii) It is injected into the trachea through the crico-thyroid membrane after local anaesthesia. General anaesthesia may be needed for children.

Propyliodone is opaque to X-rays and is of value in the diagnosis of bronchiectasis, lung abscess and new growth of the lung. About 16 ml. are required for each lung in an adult. It has the advantage over its predecessor, iodized oil ('Lipiodol'), of not remaining for long periods in the bronchi and alveoli.

DRUGS ACTING ON THE NOSE AND NASAL SINUSES

While it is not possible to give in detail all the drugs which are employed in affections of the nose, the following are the most important methods of application.

Nasal Drops (*Naristillae*)

The most well known are ephedrine nasal drops which have a vaso-constricting action and thereby help to shrink swollen and congested mucous membrane. They are of value in hay fever, sinusitis and also in acute otitis media where they decongest the mucous membrane around the opening of the Eustachian tube and allow drainage from the middle ear.

Oily solutions should not be instilled into the nose as they interfere with the action of cilia, and liquid paraffin may cause lipoid pneunionic.

Drops should be instilled with the patient lying down with the head extended and breathing through the mouth.

Many proprietary nasal decongestants are available, e.g. 'Endrine', 'Neophryn', 'Privine', 'Otrivine'.

Nasal douches (*Collunaria*)

Various solutions including saline and alkaline lotions are employed for cleansing the nose of copious discharge and crusts.

They are best given with a douche can or funnel attached to an appropriate length of rubber tubing. The height of the can should not be more than 30 cm (12 inches) above the patient's head. During the procedure the patient should be instructed to breathe heavily through the mouth.

The use of the Higginson syringe is most undesirable on account of the dangerously high pressure which can be obtained. Fluid may thus be forced into the middle ear via the Eustachian tube, causing a spread of infection.

Sniffing solutions into the nasal cavity is also inadvisable and may be followed by headache.

Nasal sprays (*Nebulae*)

Watery solutions are employed and sprayed into the nasal cavities by an appropriate atomizer or used as nasal drops.

Ephedrine, xylometazoline ('Otrivine') and 'Tuamine sulphate' are used for catarrhal affections of the nose and for nasal sinusitis. These substances are preferable to others (e.g. adrenaline and naphazoline), which cause severe "rebound" congestion of the nasal mucosa.

Inhalations

Inhalations of menthol, 120 mg, 2 grains (4 or 5 small crystals), also menthol and benzoin and menthol and eucalyptus or compound tincture of benzoin (*Tinctura benzoini composita*—Friar's balsam), 4 ml. (60 minims) to 500 ml. (1 pint) of boiling water, are commonly employed. They are of value in sinusitis, acute nasal catarrh, laryngitis, tracheitis and bronchitis.

Some drugs may be given by inhalation because they are absorbed from the respiratory tract, e.g. ergotamine inhalation in an aerosol spray used in migraine.

Insufflations and snuffs

These are occasionally employed, a special powder insufflator being used in some cases.

    e.g. Orthocaine ('Orthoform') or benzocaine ('Anaesthesin') for pain.

    Menthol snuff for nasal catarrh.

    Posterior pituitary snuff ('Disipidin') for diabetes insipidus.

Local anaesthetics

Injections of procaine ('Novocain') ½ per cent, with a few drops of adrenaline, 1 in 1000, may be used.

E

Cocaine (5 to 10 per cent), which is never injected, may be used to produce local anaesthesia by plugging the nasal cavity with strips of 1·5 cm. (½-inch) gauze soaked in the solution.

Cocaine ointment may also be applied on a wool-coated probe.

'Decicain' (amethocaine), 2 per cent, is sometimes used instead of cocaine. Amethocaine has even been made into "Lollipops" for use before bronchoscopy!

Caustics

Chromic acid, trichloracetic acid, silver nitrate or the electric cautery may be applied to ulcers in the nasal mucous membrane; or to a bleeding-point to stop epistaxis.

DRUGS APPLIED TO THE LARYNX

Various drugs are applied to the larynx by inhalations, insufflations and sprays.

Inhalations

Menthol and Friar's balsam are used as in the treatment of nasal conditions.

Sprays

Sprays containing menthol and camphor may be used for laryngitis. Lignocaine, 2 ml. of a 4 per cent solution, may be sprayed onto the larynx after the pharynx has been rendered insensitive by sucking a lozenge containing 150 mg benzocaine in order to produce anaesthesia for bronchoscopy.

CHAPTER 10

Drugs Acting on the Urinary System

The urinary system is formed by the kidneys, ureters, bladder and urethra. The kidneys are excretory glands and consist of cortex and medulla which are made up of Malpigian bodies and tubules. The ureter, its upper expanded part of the pelvis, the bladder and urethra form the ducts and reservoir via which the urine reaches the exterior.

The processes employed by the kidneys in the formation of urine are:

1. Filtration of water and salts through the Malpighian bodies.

2. Secretion of various substances by the tubules.

3. Absorption of water and substances excreted by the first two processes but required by the body to maintain the composition of the blood at a constant level.

The primary function of the kidneys is to keep the composition of the blood constant by:

(i) The excretion of water.

(ii) The excretion of the end products of protein metabolism.

(iii) The excretion of salts.

(iv) The excretion of drugs, toxins and chemical substances which may be harmful.

The kidneys are therefore of great importance in dealing with the subject of drugs. Many drugs given internally by mouth or injection, are excreted by the kidneys either in their original form or else changed by chemical action in the body (e.g. by the liver).

Some of these drugs have no effect on the urinary tract; others have a beneficial action in certain conditions and are given for this action. Finally, some have a harmful effect, especially when used in toxic doses, and may produce serious urinary symptoms such as haematuria.

Diseases of the urinary tract

These include congenital abnormalities, traumatic and mechanical conditions, acute or chronic inflammation of the kidneys (nephritis), of the pelvis (pyelitis), of the bladder (cystitis), and of the urethra (urethritis), tuberculosis and new growths. Abnormal products of metabolism may also be excreted in the urine. Medical treatment may be required for many of these conditions. Further, it may be necessary to modify the excretory functions of the kidneys in order to relieve symptoms caused by disease of other organs, e.g. the removal of fluid in cases of oedema.

DRUGS INCREASING THE OUTPUT OF URINE (DIURETICS)

A diuretic is a substance which increases the output of urine. These agents act on the kidneys and increase the output of water and also certain electrolytes such as sodium and bicarbonate.

The amount of urine normally excreted depends on three factors:
(i) The fluid intake.
(ii) The fluid lost by the evaporation of sweat.
(iii) The amount lost via the bowel.

The most obvious physiological diuretic is water. In many cases, when the kidneys are normal this is the most suitable method of producing an increased urinary flow. On the other hand, diuretics are given in order to get rid of surplus fluid already present in the body, i.e. oedema. This occurs when water and salt are retained in the body particularly in the following conditions:

(*a*) congestive heart failure, (*b*) pulmonary oedema and congestion, (*c*) ascites in cirrhosis of the liver, (*d*) nephrotic syndrome.

The processes employed by the kidneys in the formation of urine have already been mentioned. A diuretic may act in one of the following ways:

(i) Increasing the filtration of water and salts through the Malpighian bodies by generally improving the blood supply to the kidneys. Blood transfusion and saline infusions will do this in cases of surgical shock and dehydration. Digitalis will improve the renal circulation in cardiac failure, especially when due to atrial fibrillation.

(ii) By preventing the reabsorption of water in the renal tubules, e.g. urea.

(iii) By preventing the reabsorption of salts by the renal tubules thereby ensuring an increased excretion especially of sodium. The most effective and important diuretics, e.g. the thiazides, act in this way.

In addition to prescribing diuretics to reduce oedema it may be necessary to restrict salt intake. Less often it is necessary to restrict fluid intake also. In contrast to the increased sodium excretion, which is one of the objects of administering diuretics, there is increased potassium loss. This may result in general muscular weakness, especially in the nephrotic syndrome and cirrhosis of the liver. To counteract this potassium supplements are often required. To assess this periodic estimations of the blood electrolytes may be needed.

The drugs used as diuretics may be classified thus:

I. The major diuretics.

(*a*) Mercurial diuretics, e.g. mersalyl, 'Neptal'.

(*b*) The thiazides and related compounds (non-mercurial), e.g. chlorothiazide ('Saluric'), bendrofluazide, hydrofluomethiazide, chlorthalidone ('Hygroton'), frusemide ('Lasix').

(*c*) Ethacrynic acid ('Edecrin').

(*d*) Potassium-conserving diuretics, e.g. triamterene ('Dytac'), and spironolactone ('Aldactone—A').

(*e*) Osmotic diuretics.

II. The minor diuretics.

(*a*) The saline diuretics, e.g. potassium citrate.

(*b*) Urea.

(*c*) Diuretics of the caffeine group.

(*d*) Cardiac diuretics, e.g. digitalis.

The major diuretics are the only ones in general use in the treatment of the severe oedema of congestive heart failure and the other conditions mentioned above.

I. THE MAJOR DIURETICS

(a) Mercurial diuretics e.g. Mersalyl, 'Neptal'

For many years these were the only powerful diuretics available but with the advent of newer drugs they are now infrequently used. They are complicated organic compounds of mercury and are given by deep intramuscular injection, care being taken to avoid any subcutaneous injection which is liable to cause sloughing of the tissues. Intravenous injection is also very dangerous and may cause fatal collapse. In any case it is usual to give a test dose of 0·5 ml. before the full dose of 2 ml. is given the following morning. Mercury is slowly excreted so that as a rule not more than two injections weekly are given.

The thiazides and related compounds

Chlorothiazide ('Saluric'). 500 to 2000 mg (2 G) daily.

This, together with a number of drugs which have a similar basic chemical composition, is a very potent non-mercurial diuretic which is administered by mouth. The effect of 2 grams is equivalent to that of 2 ml. of mersalyl injection. It acts on the renal tubules causing an increased excretion of water, sodium and to a lesser extent of potassium.

It may be given on alternate days or for the first three or four consecutive days in any one week. One gram is given between 6 and 8 a.m. and 1 gram between 12 noon and 2 p.m. in order that the main diuresis may occur before the patient goes to sleep. Later these doses may be reduced to 0·5 gram.

In view of the possibility of potassium depletion it is advisable to give at least 1 gram of potassium chloride daily at the same time when the course of treatment is prolonged.

Other thiazides in use are hydrochlorothiazide ('Hydrosaluric'), bendrofluazide ('Neo-Naclex'), hydroflumethiazide ('Hydrenox') and cyclopenthiazide ('Navidrex').

Chlorthalidone ('Hygroton') is less likely to cause potassium loss and only one morning dose of 100 to 200 mg on alternate days or twice weekly is necessary.

Frusemide ('Lasix') is a powerful diuretic given in doses of 40 to 200 mg daily, by mouth.

Ethacrynic acid ('Edecrin')

This is a powerful diuretic not related chemically to the others (dose: 50 to 200 mg daily).

Frusemide and ethacrynic acid both have a rapid onset and short duration of action. Oral doses act for 2 to 4 hours. Diuresis commences almost immediately after an intravenous injection of one of these drugs (frusemide 20 to 40 mg, ethacrynic acid 25 to

50 mg), which are therefore valuable in the emergency treatment of pulmonary oedema.

All of the diuretics so far described cause loss of potassium in the urine and, in the case of the non-mercurial diuretics, serious potassium deficiency may result. The patient should therefore eat potassium-rich foods, such as oranges, every day. A potassium supplement such as 'Slow-K' (two to six 600-mg tablets daily) is usually necessary, however, with the non-mercurial diuretics.

Chlorothiazide and the allied drugs increase the action of hypotensive drugs so that the dose of these must be reduced if one happens to be used at the same time otherwise an excessive fall in blood pressure may be caused. Sensitivity to the action of digitalis may also be increased by the potassium deficiency induced by these diuretics.

(d) Potassium-conserving diuretics

By themselves, these are weak diuretics but when they are used in combination with a thiazide a powerful diuretic effect is obtained. Renal tubular loss of potassium is inhibited and the need for potassium supplements is abolished or reduced.

The drugs in this group are:

Triamterine ('Dytac'). Dose: 150 to 250 mg daily in divided doses. It is unrelated to the other diuretics.

Spironolactone ('Aldactone-A'). Dose: 25 to 50 mg q.d.s. This drug is an *aldosterone-antagonist* and is useful in cases where there is excessive secretion of the hormone aldosterone by the adrenal gland (hyperaldosteronism). This may occur as a secondary phenomonon in very severe congestive cardiac failure or in cirrhosis of the liver, for example. The secondary aldosteronism makes the oedema or ascites worse since the action of aldosterone is to cause reabsorption of sodium in the distal renal tubule. Water is retained in the body with the sodium. Spironolactone antagonizes the sodium-retaining and potassium-losing effect of aldosterone.

Amiloride ('Midamor'). Dose: 5 to 20 mg daily.

(e) Osmotic diuretics e.g. Mannitol

Intravenous hypertonic mannitol given to patients with healthy kidneys can produce a large diuresis. This may be useful in the treatment of some cases of poisoning to hasten the excretion of a drug overdose.

Acetazolamide ('Diamox') is not a powerful diuretic and is mainly used in the treatment of glaucoma.

II. THE MINOR DIURETICS

(a) The saline diuretics

Potassium citrate (4 grams, 15 to 60 grains), in addition to turning the urine alkaline, has a mild diuretic effect.

(b) Urea

Urea, which is normally present in the blood and excreted in the urine, acts as a diuretic if additional large doses are given by mouth, e g. 1 gram (15 grains) in 60 ml. of water, three times daily.

(c) Diuretics of the caffeine group

Caffeine (*Caffeina*)

This is an alkaloid which has diuretic properties. In addition it stimulates the nervous system, causing wakefulness and increased mental activity. In medicinal doses it also stimulates the vasomotor centre and the heart muscle to some extent. It is present in small quantities in coffee which explains the mildly stimulating and diuretic effect of this beverage. Preparations include:

Caffeine (*Caffeina*), 300 mg (2 to 5 grains).
Caffeine citrate (*Caffeinae citras*) 600 mg (2 to 10 grains).

(d) Cardiac diuretics

It has already been explained that digitalis acts as a diuretic in heart disease by reason of the improvement of the general circulation which, in turn, increases the blood supply to the kidneys. It is, of course, of special value in cases of heart failure, with oedema due to atrial fibrillation. It does not increase the urinary output in normal persons.

Methods of reducing general oedema

One of the causes of generalized oedema is the retention of sodium within the body which, in turn, causes the retention of an excess of fluid in the tissues.

In treating such cases the following methods are employed:

1. Diuretics to increase fluid output by the kidneys.
2. Restricted sodium intake (salt-free diet).
3. Restricted fluid intake.
4. The use of cation exchange resins.
5. Peritoneal dialysis with a solution containing 6.36% dextrose.

Cation exchange resins are substances which prevent the absorption of sodium from the alimentary canal and which can, therefore, be used to assist the effects of the other forms of therapy, e.g. 'Katonium', average dose 15 grams twice daily with meals. It is important to check the blood electrolytes during their use.

Other methods of removing surplus fluid from the body include:
Paracentesis thoracis.
Paracentesis abdominis.
Southey's tubes, inserted into oedematous legs.
Incision on the dorsum of the oedematous feet.

DRUGS RENDERING THE URINE ALKALINE

The urine is normally slightly acid in reaction, i.e. it turns blue litmus red.

In addition to this method of indicating the reaction of urine (or any other liquid), the reaction may also be stated in terms of what is called the hydrogen-ion concentration or pH. A solution which is neutral is described as having a pH of 7. Acid solutions have a pH of less than 7 (e.g. pH 5) while alkaline solutions have a pH greater than 7 (e.g. pH 9). Special indicators are required to determine pH accurately.

It is frequently desirable to render the urine alkaline, for example to hinder the growth of organisms, especially the *Escherichia coli*, which does not flourish in alkaline urine. Alkalis are therefore given in cases of pyelitis and cystitis, particularly in the acute stages. Strongly acid urine is also irritating to the bladder and in some cases may cause frequent and painful micturition.

Alkalis, usually given in mixture form, include:

Potassium citrate (*Potassii citras*) ⎫
Sodium citrate (*Sodii citras*) ⎬ 4 grams,
Sodium bicarbonate (*Sodii bicarbonas*) ⎭ (5 to 60 grains)

DRUGS RENDERING THE URINE ACID

Drugs are occasionally given to make the urine acid in order to permit the efficient action of other drugs which are only effective in an acid medium. For example, mandelic acid and its preparations are only effective as urinary antiseptics against the *Escherichia coli* in acid urine (pH 5·5).

The following salts are used:

Acid sodium phosphate (*Sodii phosphas acidus*), 16 grams (30 to 240 grains).

URINARY ANTISEPTICS

Urinary antiseptics are drugs which, when given by mouth, are excreted by the kidneys and have the power of inhibiting the growth of organisms in the urine. The most important urinary antiseptics are:

Sulphonamides. Antibiotics.

The sulphonamides

In addition to their action on streptococcal, pneumococcal, meningococcal and other infections in various parts of the body, drugs of this group are of special value in infections of the urinary tract due to the *Escherichia coli*. They are, therefore, used in the treatment of pyelitis and cystitis. They are also effective against the gonococcus (p. 228). Most soluble sulphonamides act as urinary antiseptics. **Sulphamethizole** ('Urolucosil'), 100–200 mg every four hours, is specially employed for this purpose.

Sulphonamides act by interfering with synthesis of folate in bacteria. Bacteria have to synthesize their own folate because they cannot absorb it from their environment. Folate is necessary for the growth of bacteria and sulphonamides therefore stop them from growing. Sulphonamides are thus said to have a *bacteriostatic* action. Another drug has been made specifically to block the next step in bacterial folate metabolism, in case the organism overcomes the action of the sulphonamide. This recently developed synthetic antibacterial drug is called trimethoprin. It too is bacteriostatic when used alone. When used together with a sulphonamide, however, the effect of the combination is *bactericidal*. 'Septrin' and 'Bactrim' are combinations (mixtures) of sulphamethoxazole and trimethoprin. The usual dose is two tablets twice daily for adults and children over 12 years.

Antibiotics

Various antibiotics may be used depending on the organism present in the urine and its sensitivity, especially if it is unaffected by sulphonamides. Streptomycin is useful in special cases, but it must be remembered that *Escherichia coli* is insensitive to penicillin. Ampicillin is a useful antiobiotic for urinary tract infection (see p. 237).

Other urinary antiseptics

Nitrofurantoin ('Furadantin'), 5–8 mg per kilo body weight. This substance is active both against Gram-positive and Gram-negative organisms, including staphylococci and *B. proteus*. The average adult dose is 100 mg four times daily, with meals or milk (since it is a gastric irritant). Rarely, neuritis may follow its use.

Nalidixic acid ('Negram') 1 G six-hourly, is bactericidal to many Gram-negative organisms found in urinary tract infections. It may give a false positive test for sugar in the urine.

Mandelic acid

Mandelic acid or one of its preparations acts as a urinary antiseptic when excreted into the urine. It is essential, however, to have a certain degree of acidity present which is measured, not by litmus, but by a special indicator recording the hydrogen-ion concentration or pH. This should not exceed 5·5.

'Mandelamine' is a proprietary preparation.

The treatment of cystitis and pyelitis (summary)

Although there are various methods available, the one very commonly employed is to give sodium or potassium citrate in sufficient doses to render the urine alkaline, together with one of the sulphonamide drugs for 5 or 6 days. If it is unsuccessful, one of the other methods may then be tried. It is most important to ascertain the nature of the infecting organism, and its sensitivity.

DRUGS ACTING ON THE BLADDER

The urinary antiseptics and alkalis already mentioned are given by mouth in cases of cystitis. Hyoscyamus may be included in alkaline mixtures because it has a sedative action on the bladder and helps to relieve the symptoms of frequent or painful micturition.

Local applications are also used for washing out the bladder, particularly in cases of chronic cystitis and after operations involving the bladder.

One litre of fluid at a temperature of 110°F from a bottle about 1 metre (3 feet) above the patient is generally employed, e.g.:

Sodium bicarbonate (1 to 2 per cent).
Dilute acetic acid ($\frac{1}{2}$ per cent).
Oxycyanide of mercury (1 in 4000).
Potassium permanganate (1 in 4000).
Silver nitrate (1 in 10,000, increasing to 1 in 2000).
'Noxyflex' (2·5 per cent).

Drugs such as carbachol have an action on the muscle of the bladder causing it to contract and may be useful in the treatment of postoperative retention of urine.

Emepronium bromide ('Cetiprin') may be of value in treating an "irritable" bladder, especially after prostatectomy or radiotherapy and may relieve frequency and incontinence in the elderly. Dose: 200 mg three times a day.

DRUGS ACTING ON THE URETHRA

The main condition requring treatment is urethritis, which is usually due to the gonococcus but may be due to other causes.

Intramuscular injection of a single dose of procaine penicillin, 600,000 units, or streptomycin 1G, may be effective. Other antibiotics may be given orally.

Local applications are sometimes employed, e.g. urethral irrigations with potassium permanganate, 1 in 8000.

In order to produce local anaesthesia of the urethra, 2% lignocaine jelly ('Xylocaine gel') is used.

DRUGS USED IN THE DIAGNOSIS OF URINARY CONDITIONS

The efficiency of the kidneys may be investigated by testing their power of excreting various substances.

1. Urea

Urea is normally excreted by the kidneys and the urine contains approximately 2 per cent.

Urea concentration test. No fluid is taken for several hours, the bladder is then emptied and the patient given 15 grams of urea by mouth dissolved in 100 ml. of water. The urine is collected 1 and 2 hours later. The amount of urea in each specimen is then estimated. If the concentrating power of the kidneys is normal, the first specimen should contain at least 1·5 per cent and the second 2 per cent of urea.

Urea clearance test. There are several methods of performing this test, which depends on comparing the blood urea with the output of urea in the urine.

2. Creatinine

This is a breakdown product of the creatine found in muscle. It is freely filtered by the kidney and its clearance from the plasma can be determined by a simple formula. The creatinine clearance provides an approximate estimate of the glomemlar filtration rate (GFR). This indicates how much renal tissue is functioning.

Creatinine clearance is determined from the plasma creatinine concentration and from the urinary excretion of creatinine. Urine is collected over a timed period, preferably of 24 hours. As with all tests involving a 24-hour urine collection, the nurse should ensure that at the start of the test (e.g. at 9 a.m.) the bladder is emptied and the urine is discarded. *All* urine passed during the next 24 hours is collected in a bottle. The patient must be *asked* to empty his bladder into the bottle at the end of the test (e.g. at 9 a.m. the following day) to complete the collection.

3. Dyes

Various dyes given by intramuscular or intravenous injection are excreted by the kidneys and colour the urine (p. 46).

By passing ureteric catheters after cystoscopy, the urine from each kidney can be collected separately and the time taken for the dye to appear in the urine from each kidney can be estimated. A delay will indicate damage to one or both kidneys.

The dyes used include:

Indigocarmine, intramuscular, 50 to 100 mg.
  intravenous, 8 to 16 mg.
Methylene blue, intramuscular, 1 ml. of 5% solution.

4. Radio-opaque substances

An outline of the urinary tract obtained by X-rays after the introduction of a radio-opaque substance is called a pyelogram. This may be obtained in the following ways.

(a) Excretion or intravenous pyelography
The intravenous injection of:
Sodium diatrizoate ('Hypaque') 45 or 65% (25% for children).
Sodium metrizoate ('Triosil') 60 or 75%.
'Urografin' 76% (a mixture of diatrizoates).
Diodone ('Uriodone') 35%.
Iodoxyl ('Uropac') 75%.
These iodine-containing substances are excreted by the kidneys and, being opaque to X-rays, radiograms taken 5, 10, 30 and 50 minutes after injection show the outline of the pelvis of the kidneys, the ureters and the bladder.

Diodone is sometimes given subcutaneously with hyalase but iodoxyl is not used in this manner because it is too irritating. When given intravenously care must be taken that none of the fluid escapes from the vein or a painful arm will result.

(b) Instrumental or retrograde pyelography

A cystoscope is passed and the orifices of the ureters in the bladder determined. After a catheter has been introduced into one or both ureters, 5 to 10 ml. of sterile, 12·5 per cent solution of sodium iodide or 45% 'Hypaque' are injected, the injection ceasing when the patient complains of pain in the loin. The solution is opaque to X-rays and in this way the outline of the pelvis of the kidney is obtained.

DRUGS ALTERING THE COLOUR OF THE URINE

Normal urine is described as straw-coloured, amber or like pale sherry. The following abnormalities of colour may occur:

Bright yellow: due to santonin in acid urine.

Pink or red: due to rhubarb, senna, phenolphthalein, 'Dorbanex' or phenindione.

Black or brown: due to bile, poisoning with phenol or lysol. Rarely the urine of patients taking methyldopa may darken on exposure to air.

Blue or green: due to methylene blue.

CHAPTER 11

Drugs Acting on the Nervous System

The nervous system may be divided into three main portions:
1. The brain and spinal cord or central nervous system.
2. The nerves or peripheral nervous system.
3. The involuntary (sympathetic and autonomic) system.

The functioning elements of the system are different types of nerve cells and their fibres.

Nerve cells and fibres are sensitive to the action of various drugs which reach them via the blood and the cerebrospinal fluid. Their activities may either be stimulated, depressed or altered in function by the action of drugs.

DRUGS WHICH DEPRESS THE CENTRAL NERVOUS SYSTEM

One of the features of a number of drugs, which in full doses have the effect of depressing the nervous system, is that in small doses they often have an apparently stimulating action. This is shown for example, in the exhilarating effect of small or moderate doses of alcohol and in the excitement stage manifested during the induction of general anaesthesia.

It may be that in small doses such substances do have an initial stimulating effect. However, it must be remembered that the highest centres of the brain, namely those which are concerned with consciousness and behaviour, are the first to be affected and, normally, these centres exercise a restraining influence on the activities of an individual. It is, therefore, much more likely that these drugs exercise their depressing effect from the commencement and that the apparent stimulation is merely the result of removing the controlling action of the higher centres.

As the dosage of such drugs is increased, other centres or levels of nervous activity are depressed. Sensation is dulled, consciousness is lost, the cough and vomiting reflexes are abolished. Finally, in toxic doses, the vital centres such as the respiratory and vasomotor centres are affected, and if these are completely paralysed death ensues.

From the point of view of therapeutics these drugs may be divided into the following groups:

I. Hypnotics or drugs used to produce sleep or a general dulling of mental activity.

II. Analgesics

(a) Simple analgesics, e.g. aspirin.

(b) Analgesics with hypnotic properties, e.g. morphine.

III. Psychotropic drugs. There are two main groups of these drugs:

(a) tranquillizers which are used to relieve anxiety.

(b) those used to treat depression.

IV. Drugs which stimulate the nervous system.

V. Anticonvulsants used in the treatment of epilepsy.

VI. Drugs used in the treatment of Parkinson's disease.

VII. Drugs used in the treatment of migraine.

VIII. A miscellaneous group some of which are used in the treatment of special symptoms.

I. HYPNOTICS

In some respects it is difficult to divide hypnotics and analgesics into separate groups, for there are a number of the former which have analgesic properties as well. When given in ordinary doses they can be classified as:

Drugs having hypnotic effects only.

Drugs having analgesic effects only.

Drugs having both hypnotic and analgesic effects. The last group consists of individual drugs and preparations made by mixing drugs of the first two types.

DRUGS HAVING HYPNOTIC EFFECTS ONLY

A hypnotic or narcotic drug is one which is used to induce sleep and also has a calming or sedative action on the nervous system. It is, in fact, a substance which the lay person regards as a "drug". An analgesic relieves pain. Substances having both actions are therefore used especially to treat insomnia or sleeplessness when the patient is unable to sleep on account of pain. They may also be used to relieve severe pain irrespective of their narcotic effects, e.g. morphine. For minor degrees of pain a simple analgesic, such as aspirin, is usually all that is required.

Drug addiction. Great care and discrimination must be exercised in the use of these drugs. Many are "habit-forming"; that is, the patient feels unable to do without them. Others, if given over a period, result in a serious craving for the drug when it is withdrawn. Drug addiction is a very difficult condition to cure and sufferers will often go to extremes in order to obtain the drug and satisfy their cravings. For this reason the sale and issue of most of the drugs of this type is controlled by the Dangerous Drugs Act and they can only be obtained on a doctor's prescription (p. 6).

Insomnia. The inability to secure sufficient sleep, or failure to obtain sound restful sleep, is a problem which frequently presents itself for treatment, and it is not solved by simply prescribing one of the many available hypnotic drugs.

The first step is to ascertain, if possible, the underlying cause. A simple method of grouping cases is:

1. Primary—where no physical cause can be found, e.g. anxiety states, hysteria.

2. Secondary—where pain, physical discomfort such as in-digestion—irritation of the skin (pruritus)—frequency of micturition —cough—or some organic disease, is the cause.

In the second group, treatment is given for the underlying cause and its symptoms before, or at the same time as, active measures are adopted to procure sleep.

General management

A careful history of the patient's habits must be obtained so that any undesirable factors or contributory causes may be eliminated.

1. He should sleep in a quiet room, adequately ventilated but kept at an even temperature. The blinds should be drawn, doors and windows wedged to prevent rattling and clocks removed. (Occasionally the monotonous ticking of a clock is an aid to drowsiness.)

2. The bed-clothes should be light but warm. As a rule, a spring mattress is best, but it is not always wise to change the type of bed to which the patient is accustomed.

3. A warm bath on retiring promotes sleep in some individuals. A hot-water bottle or bed-socks are often of value, especially if coldness of the extremities is noticed.

4. Overloading the stomach shortly before bed-time is undesirable and a light evening meal is often preferable to a heavy
dinner. In such circumstances, soup, Bovril, hot milk or a preparation such as Ovaltine may be taken just before retiring, or
during the night if the patient wakes, provided it is kept hot in a
Thermos flask and the patient does not have to rouse himself to
prepare it.

5. Tea and coffee at night should be avoided. The effect of
alcohol is variable. In some patients, whisky or brandy in hot or
cold water is of great value as a night-cap while in others it produces wakefulness. Before prescribing it the possibility of producing
an alcohol habit must be considered, especially if the patient is of
an unbalanced psychological order.

6. Patients who complain of wakefulness on account of excessive
mental activity on retiring, should pass their evenings quietly and
games such as competitive cards should be avoided. Quiet reading
of unsensational literature may be recommended, while the effect
of a walk, but not vigorous exercise, before bed-time may be tried.

7. Many people sleep best on their right side; some prefer one
pillow, others like a number, and a few imagine they sleep best with
their beds in some definite position, e.g. placed north and south.

8. The patient often fears the consequences of insomnia more
than the lack of sleep, a dread which in itself may produce an
anxiety state. Reassurance is, therefore, of great importance. He
should be told that life will not be lost on this account nor will he
lose his reason.

It is clearly wrong to attempt to force the patient to sleep with
potent drugs without first attempting to remove the underlying
cause. Drugs may be essential in cases of this type in order to obtain
the tranquillity of mind necessary for psychotherapy to be effective.
They are also valuable in breaking the "habit of insomnia" which
is prone to exist in this type of case.

The fact of taking a drug is a powerful suggestive force which
will aid in procuring sleep and, in the first instance, the preparation
employed should be strong enough to produce the desired effect.
The dose and potency should subsequently be reduced without the
knowledge of the patient.

The hypnotic drugs not having any special analgesic action are:
1. The barbiturates.
2. Chloral hydrate and dichloralphenazone ('Welldorm').
3. Paraldehyde.

4. The bromides.

5. Drugs of the urea and sulphone groups.

6. Synthetic drugs such as glutethimide ('Doriden'), methyprylone ('Noludar'), methaqualone ('Mandrax'), Nitrazepam ('Mogadon') which also act as tranquillizers in smaller doses.

N.B.—Very few drugs have really proved superior to barbiturates and chloral hydrate except in special circumstances.

1. The barbiturates

There are a large number of drugs derived from barbituric acid which have a depressing effect on the central nervous system and are used as hypnotics. They have little effect on pain and are for this reason often combined with analgesic drugs in proprietary preparations.

In addition to their use as hypnotics and general sedatives in anxiety states, certain of them, e.g. phenobarbitone, are employed in the treatment of epilepsy to depress the irritability of the cerebrum.

Although a patient taking barbiturates regularly for insomnia may not be able to sleep properly without them and may come to rely on them, and they are, in this sense, habit-forming; they do not tend to produce the craving which may follow the habitual use of drugs like opium, morphine and cocaine. Some patients do, however, habitually take relatively large doses of barbiturates. In such instances sudden withdrawal may result in fits.

It is not uncommon to find cases in which an overdose has been taken either accidentally or with suicidal intent.

Barbiturates should never be used in combination with alcohol or methyl pentynol ('Oblivon') as the drugs have a cumulative effect if taken together. This is most dangerous for car drivers.

The most important barbiturates fall into three main groups, viz.:

1. Short action (3 to 6 hours) rapid excretion, e.g.:

		Dose: mg	grains
Quinalbarbitone	'Seconal'	200	$\frac{3}{4}$ to 3
Hexobarbitone	'Evipan'	500	4 to 8
Cyclobarbitone	'Phanodorm'	400	3 to 6

2. Intermediate action (4 to 8 hours), e.g.:

Amylobarbitone	'Amytal'	300	$1\frac{1}{2}$ to 5
Pentobarbitone	'Nembutal'	200	1 to 3
Butobarbitone	'Soneryl'	200	1 to 3

3. Long acting (8 to 16 hours), e.g.:

		Dose: mg	grains
Phenobarbitone	'Luminal'	120	$\frac{1}{2}$ to 2
Methyl phenobarbitone	'Prominal'	200	1 to 3

Among the many other drugs containing barbiturates are 'Carbrital', 'Sonalgin', 'Evidorm'. 'Tuinal' (a mixture of quinalbarbitone and amylobarbitone).

The sodium preparations of the various barbiturates are more soluble than the other forms and act more quickly. Soluble phenobarbitone (sodium) may be given by intramuscular injection (200 mg, 3 grains).

Symptoms of barbiturate poisoning include:

Increasing coma.

Depression of the respiratory centre with slow, shallow breathing.

Abolition of the tendon and eye reflexes.

Fall in blood pressure.

Later, bronchopneumonia.

Treatment of barbiturate poisoning

1. *Ensure a clear airway and adequate ventilation.* Endotracheal intubation and perhaps the use of a mechanical ventilator may be necessary.

2. *Gastric lavage* should be performed if less than four hours have elapsed since the overdose was taken.

3. In the more severe cases, active measures must be taken to aid the elimination of the drug from the body. This may be done by forced diuresis or by haemodialysis ('artificial kidney').

Forced diuresis is feasible if the patient is without cardiac or renal disease. Large volumes of normal saline and 5% dextrose solution, specified quantities of sodium bicarbonate and potassium chloride, and a slow drip of 20% mannitol solution (500 ml. over 12 hours) are administered intravenously. A careful watch is kept on the patient's clinical condition, fluid balance and serum electrolytes.

Haemodialysis is indicated if the initial blood barbiturate level is greater than 15 mg/100 ml. in the case of long-acting barbiturates or 4 mg/100 ml. in the case of intermediate-acting barbiturates. It is also indicated if the blood level of barbiturate continues to rise or the clinical condition deteriorates in spite of forced diuresis.

Barbiturates should be used with special caution in:
1. Allergic patients (asthma, angio-neurotic oedema).
2. Defective renal or hepatic function.
3. Diabetes.
4. Thyrotoxicosis.
5. Old age.

The tendency to habit formation may be greatly diminished by withholding from the patient the knowledge of the name and dose of the drug he is taking.

2. Chloral hydrate (*Chloral hydras*), 0·3 to 2 grams (5 to 30 grains).

This is a drug which occurs in crystalline form but is usually dissolved in water and given in the form of a mixture or draught, but its bitter flavour is not easy to conceal.

Chloral hydrate 1·2 gram (20 grains) with 1 ml. (15 minims) of tincture of opium is a useful hypnotic.

Another preparation is syrup of chloral (*Syrupus chloralis*). This is sometimes used for children, but a serious word of warning must be given. Although the official dose of the syrup is up to 8 ml. (30 to 120 minims), this is an adult dose, and 4 ml. (60 minims) contain about 700 mg (11 grains) of chloral. This is a very large and dangerous dose for a child, even though infants tolerate chloral well. A suitable dose for an infant of 1 year is 120 mg (2 grains) i.e. not more than 1 ml. (15 minims) of syrup of chloral.

Chloral is a very effective hypnotic, especially for children and the elderly, which does not predispose to habit formation. It is quite safe to give to cardiac patients in ordinary doses, although at one time this was thought to be inadvisable.

'Welldorm' is a proprietary tablet or elixir containing dichloral-phenazone which avoids the bitter taste of mixtures.

3. Paraldehyde (*Paraldehydum*), oral dose 2 to 8 ml.

This is a colourless liquid with a characteristic pungent odour and unpleasant taste which should be stored in the dark. It is, however, a very safe and valuable hypnotic. Its duration of action is relatively short and it is excreted in the breath so that it can be smelt some hours after its administration.

Paraldehyde is now usually given by intramuscular injection (*Injectio paraldehydi*, dose, 5 to 10 ml.) but a plastic syringe must not be used.

It is sometimes prescribed in mixture form for oral administration, but is only slightly soluble in water. The bottle must be carefully shaken as the bulk of the paraldehyde tends to float on the top of the mixture.

It can also be given per rectum, when double the oral dose may be ordered.

Accidents have sometimes happened, and proved fatal, because the dose of paraldehyde has been misread. It must be emphasized that the dose of pure paraldehyde is measured in minims, drachms or millilitres; and only when previously mixed with water will the dose be ordered as one or more ounces. The nurse must always make quite certain which of the two she is using.

4. Synthetic drugs. e.g. (*a*) Methaqualone ('Mandrax') (dose 250 mg) which should not be given to patients with liver disease and alcohol should be avoided, (*b*) Nitrazepam ('Mogadon) (dose 5 mg). This should not be taken in early pregnancy or with alcohol.

5. The bromides

Bromides are crystalline salts which are soluble in water, e.g.

Potassium bromide (*Potassii bromidum*)	
Sodium bromide (*Sodii bromidum*)	0·3 to 2 grams
Ammonium bromide (*Ammonii bromidum*)	5 to 30 grains.

They may be given in mixture form and have a general sedative effect on the nervous system. In order to produce sleep they may be given with chloral.

Bromides have largely been replaced by barbiturates in the treatment of epilepsy and as nerve sedatives in cases of mental anxiety and states of excitement.

"Bromism" (p. 27) may develop in persons especially sensitive to bromide (idiosyncrasy) and in cases of overdosage. The symptoms include skin eruptions which resemble acne or eczema. Bromides are not well tolerated by the elderly and, therefore, should be used with caution in old age, for they are then liable to cause mental confusion. They have no special habit-forming properties but are rarely, if ever, used.

6. The urea group contains some mild and safe hypnotics, e.g.

Carbromal ('Adalin')	300–1000 mg.
Bromvaletone ('Bromural')	300–600 mg.

7. Methylpentynol ('Oblivon') is a drug which has a sedative effect and is particularly useful in allaying apprehension, nervous tension or excitement. It is given in the form of capsules or an elixir, but, being an alcohol, should not be combined with barbiturates.

II ANALGESICS

DRUGS HAVING ANALGESIC EFFECTS (ANODYNES)

The most important drugs of this type are:

Acetylsalicylic acid (*Acidum acetylsalicylicum*—Aspirin), 300–1000 mg (5–15 grains).

When given by mouth this drug is of great value in relieving minor degrees of pain and discomfort. It also induces sweating and tends to lower the body temperature, i.e. it is also an antipyretic (p. 57). Like sodium salicylate, it is of value in the treatment of rheumatism, chorea, neuralgia, fibrositis and gout.

It may be given in combination with barbiturates, which have hypnotic effects, while any associated pain is controlled by aspirin.

Aspirin has a slight local anaesthetic action when applied to mucous membranes and so is useful as a gargle to relieve pain after tonsillectomy 600 mg in 30 ml. (10 grains in 1 ounce) of water.

It is given either in tablets, containing 300 mg (5 grains), or in mixture form.

Calcium aspirin, known also as Aspirin Soluble Tablets, (B.P.) and 'Disprin' is more soluble than ordinary aspirin. It is therefore more readily absorbed and acts more quickly. It has less tendency to cause gastric irritation.

Tablets containing aspirin mixed with other drugs are also commonly used, e.g.

Aspirin Compound Tablets, (B.P.C.), Tab. APC, containing aspirin 225 mg ($3\frac{1}{2}$ gr.), phenacetin 150 mg ($2\frac{1}{2}$ gr.), caffeine 30 mg ($\frac{1}{2}$ gr.).

Aspirin, Phenacetin and Codeine Tablets, (B.P.), contains aspirin 250 mg (4 gr.), phenacetin 250 mg (4 gr.), codeine phosphate 8 mg ($\frac{1}{8}$ gr.).

'Veganin' is similar to the latter but contains paracetamol instead of Phenacetin.

'Anadin' contains aspirin, phenacetin, caffeine and quinine sulphate. There are many analgesic preparations, including 'Paynocil', 'Zactirin', and 'Doloxine' containing aspirin in various forms and with other drugs.

Aspirin poisoning. Accidental and suicidal aspirin poisoning are not uncommon. The symptoms include nausea, vomiting, noises in the head, rashes, and a weak, rapid pulse. Large doses cause coma and death.

Treatment: The stomach should be washed out, preferably with

5% sodium bicarbonate solution or an emetic may be given. Milk or water containing bicarbonate by mouth and intravenous fluids, e.g. sodium lactate solution, saline, Dextran or Hartmann's solution may be needed. Forced alkaline diuresis, using bicarbonate infusions, will increase the rate of urinary excretion of aspirin. An "artificial kidney" (haemodialysis) may save severe cases during the treatment of which estimations of the plasma salicylate should be made. In infants, the poison can be removed by peritoneal dialysis or by exchange transfusion. The latter is not feasible in adults because of the large volumes of donor blood required.

Vitamin K_1, 10 mg intramuscularly, is given to correct the defect in blood coagulation caused by salicylates.

Aspirin in ordinary doses sometimes causes gastric bleeding and haematemesis, owing to its irritant action on the gastric mucosa and some asthmatics are sensitive to aspirin.

Other pain relieving drugs include: Dihydrocodeine ('DF118'), 'Zactirin', 'Saridone', paracetamol ('Panadol') and mefenamic acid ('Ponstan').

Sodium salicylate (2 grams, 10 to 30 grains)

This drug is used especially in the treatment of rheumatic fever in which it reduces the temperature to normal and relieves the joint pains. Full doses must be given at first and then gradually reduced. It is usual to prescribe an equal quantity of sodium bicarbonate at the same time with a view to reducing toxic effects. The symptoms of overdosage are similar to those produced by aspirin.

Phenacetin (*Phenacetinum*), 600 mg (5 to 10 grains)

This is an analgesic drug especially used to relieve headache and minor degrees of pain. It is often combined with aspirin and caffeine and given in tablet form. Prolonged dosage may lead to serious kidney damage and it has been replaced by the safer paracetamol.

Amidopyrine acts as an analgesic and antipyretic, but in some persons who show idiosyncrasy it is liable to produce the dangerous condition known as agranulocytosis, in which the polymorphonuclear leucocytes of the blood are markedly diminished by reason of a toxic action on the bone marrow (p. 103). The drug has, therefore, fallen into disuse.

DRUGS HAVING BOTH HYPNOTIC AND ANALGESIC PROPERTIES

There are a number of drugs of this type of which opium and its alkaloid morphine are the most important. Their use is controlled by the Dangerous Drugs Act.

Opium

Opium is the dried juice of certain poppy heads which are grown mainly in China, India and Persia. It is one of the oldest of drugs and its use was known to the Egyptians, Romans and Greeks. Its activity is due to a number of alkaloids, of which the most important is morphine. Opium contains about 10 per cent of morphine and its important pharmacological actions can be attributed to this alkaloid.

Morphine, 8 to 20 mg ($\frac{1}{8}$ to $\frac{1}{3}$ grain)

Morphine acts on the central nervous system, depressing the important centres and has a special effect on the sensory nerve cells, which explains its value in the relief of pain.

(a) **Action on the higher centres.** In some persons there is at first a period of well-being or excitement after its administration due to the removal of the control of the highest centres of nervous activity (cf. anaesthetics). This is soon followed by a general dulling of perception so that the patient assumes a drowsy state with diminished power of attention. While this is going on the sensory centres are depressed and the appreciation of pain and discomfort are markedly diminished. Movements tend to become clumsy and the patient passes into a sleep from which, however, he can be easily roused but which returns when he is left undisturbed.

(b) **Action on the medulla.** The *respiratory centre* is depressed so that respiration becomes slower and shallower. A most important action of morphine. It is helpful in the treatment of dyspnoea in cases of left ventricular heart failure with pulmonary oedema.

The *cough reflex centre* is depressed and this makes opium and morphine of value in allaying irritating and useless cough.

The *vomiting centre* is affected in some persons. In such a case, small doses of morphine appear to have a contradictory action and the centre is stimulated so that the patient vomits. In larger doses the centre is depressed by morphine.

The *vasomotor centre* is somewhat depressed, but to a relatively less extent than the respiratory centre.

Eye reflexs: the pupils are contracted.

(c) **Action on the alimentary system.** The nerve plexuses in the walls of the bowel are depressed by the action of opium and morphine. This slows down peristalsis, so that constipation results and the faeces tend to become hard and dry from their prolonged stay in the gut, during which additional water is absorbed by the colon. Advantage is taken of this constipating effect in the treatment of some cases of diarrhoea, e.g. kaolin and morphine mixture.

Morphine poisoning. The depth of sleep and other effects produced are dependent on the dose of morphine or opium given. The description so far given would apply to the ordinary therapeutic doses, e.g. not exceeding 20 mg ($\frac{1}{3}$ grain) of morphine. In larger, and therefore, poisonous doses sleep develops into coma from which it is very difficult to rouse the patient. Reflexes are lost. The depression of the respiratory centre is so marked that the rate of breathing may be slowed to less than 12 per minute. The contracted pupil becomes pin-point in size. The pulse is weak.

Treatment of morphine poisoning. The general principle is to stimulate the patient in every way. Also, the stomach should be washed out with a solution of potassium permanganate, 4 grams (60 grains) in 2 gallons of water, even if the drug has been given by injection, as it is probable that some of the drug given in this way is excreted into the stomach. This may be followed by giving strong black coffee. Sometimes gastric aspiration followed by lavage with not more than 1 litre of water is preferred.

If possible, the patient should be kept awake by walking him about, flicking with wet towels, electrical stimulation, etc. If respiration has ceased, pulmonary ventilation must be maintained and some form of artificial respiration performed. In other cases, inhalations of carbon dioxide and oxygen are necessary. Injections, of nikethamide or caffeine have been used to stimulate the respiratory centre, and injections of atropine are helpful.

The antidote to morphine poisoning which should always be used is nalorphine ('Lethidrone'), a powerful stimulant of the respiratory centre, which is given in 10 mg doses intravenously. It may also be used in overdosage with pethidine and methadone ('Physeptone'). Amiphenazole ('Daptazole') has also been used.

Idiosyncrasy. Children do not tolerate morphine or opium well, and doses very small in proportion to the age should be given. This is especially important in infants.

It has been pointed out that some individuals tend to show a degree of restlessness after the injection of morphine. In others, vomiting may be severe.

Tolerance. The continued use of morphine leads to a fairly rapidly developing tolerance for the drug and larger and larger doses are required in order to produce effective results. This is probably due to the fact that the tissues acquire the ability of destroying morphine more quickly. It is, therefore, not uncommon to find cases (e.g. those suffering from inoperable carcinoma) receiving 120 mg (two or more gr.), several times a day. This amount has been reached by increasing the dose gradually over a period of weeks or months. A dose of this size given to an individual unaccustomed to the drug would, of course, have very serious or fatal results.

Undesirable effects of morphine

1. *On the alimentary system.* Vomiting and constipation have already been mentioned.

2. *On the respiratory system.* Although useful in allaying cough, the fact that morphine depresses the respiratory centre necessitates great care in its employment in cases of respiratory disease, such as pneumonia (later stages), bronchitis and bronchial asthma. It should never be used in the treatment of an asthmatic attack since it can produce fatal results.

3. *Psychological effects.* Morphine is one of the most important substances responsible for drug addiction. While in the Western Hemisphere the habit of opium smoking is rare, it has not been entirely stamped out in the East in spite of recent attempts to control the evil. This habit ultimately renders the addict a nervous wreck, weak in character, with little moral sense and poor in physique.

The craving for the drug is most commonly produced in the West by its prolonged administration during a painful illness. It is, therefore, most important that it should only be used for limited periods in acute disease. Only in conditions such as inoperable carcinoma, which are likely to prove rapidly fatal, is its use justifiable in chronic disease.

The treatment of drug addiction is extremely difficult. The patient must be confined to a special institution, where attempts are made to substitute the offending drug with others in gradually decreasing doses until both have been entirely withdrawn. Relapses after treatment are common.

Legal control of morphine (p. 6).

Preparations of opium

Ipecacuanha and opium powder (*Pulvis ipecacuanhae et opii*— Dover's powder), 600 mg (5 to 10 grains).

Tincture of opium (*Tinctura opii*—laudanum), 2 ml. (5 to 30 minims).

'Nepenthe' is a proprietary preparation resembling, but more pleasant to take than tincture of opium. Dose, 2·5 ml. (20 to 40 minims).

Gall and opium ointment (*Unguentum gallae cum opio*), used in the treatment of haemorrhoids.

Preparations of morphine

Morphine sulphate injection (B.P.), 8 to 20 mg ($\frac{1}{8}$ to $\frac{1}{3}$ grain). Ampoules containing 10 mg ($\frac{1}{6}$ gr.), 15 mg ($\frac{1}{4}$ gr.), 20 mg ($\frac{1}{3}$ gr.) and 30 mg ($\frac{1}{2}$ gr.) are available.

Morphine and atropine injection (B.P.C.). Ampoules of 1 ml. contain 10 mg ($\frac{1}{6}$ gr.) of morphine and atropine 0·6 mg ($\frac{1}{100}$ gr.).

Morphine and hyoscine injection. Ampoules of 1 ml. contain morphine to 10 mg ($\frac{1}{6}$ gr.) and hyoscine 0·4 mg ($\frac{1}{150}$ gr.) approx.

Solution of morphine hydrochloride 1 per cent (*Liquor morphinae hydrochloridi*), 0·3 to 2 ml. (5 to 30 minims).

Morphine suppository (*Suppositorium morphinae*), contains 15 mg ($\frac{1}{2}$ grain).

Morphine is generally given by hypodermic injection, but can be given by mouth.

Drugs resembling morphine

Papaveretum injection. Dose, 10–20 mg ($\frac{1}{6}$ to $\frac{1}{3}$ grain). This contains alkaloids of opium and is the basis of proprietary preparations such as 'Omnopon'.

It has the analgesic and narcotic properties of morphine but produces fewer side-effects.

Papaverine (*Papaverina*), 250 mg (2 to 4 grains). This also is an alkaloid of opium, which has an antispasmodic action but little analgesic effect. Eupaverine is a similar synthetic substance which is stated to be less toxic. These two drugs must not be confused with Papaveretum, and it will be noted that the doses are different.

'Dromoran' (levorphanol), 2–3 mg, is a proprietary preparation having a similar action to morphine.

Pethidine (D.D.A.)

This is a synthetic drug which has an analgesic effect and although less powerful, may be used instead of morphine in some cases. It is very useful in obstetrics. Its duration of action is rather short and it may be necessary to administer it every three hours. Barbiturates or promazine may be given at the same time. The dose is 25–100 milligrams, either by mouth or subcutaneous injection.

The intravenous dose is 25–50 mg.

Addiction is rapidly acquired, and it may produce dizziness, nausea and sweating.

'Pethilorfan' contains pethidine, 100 mg with levallorphan, 1·25 mg in 2 ml. ampoules. The latter drug antagonizes the depressing effect of pethidine on the respiratory centre.

Methadone ('Physeptone', 'Amidone'), 5 to 10 mg, D.D.A.

This is a powerful synthetic analgesic having no sedative or hypnotic effect which may be given either by mouth, subcutaneous or intramuscular injection. It may produce minor toxic effects such as nausea, vomiting, dizziness and sweating. These are more likely to occur in ambulant patients, so that patients should remain in bed after it has been given. It is also the basis of a useful cough linctus which usually contains 2 mg of methadone in 5 ml. Children tolerate only very small doses and the linctus should be kept out of their reach.

Diamorphine (heroin), 5–10 mg, $\frac{1}{12}$ to $\frac{1}{6}$ grain (D.D.A.)

This is a drug having a similar action to morphine and is even more likely to produce addiction. Its manufacture is therefore forbidden in some countries. It may be given as an injection for the relief of pain, e.g. in myocardial infarction, but its main use is for pain in terminal conditions. It is also used in a linctus for the relief of troublesome coughs, e.g.:

Diamorphine (heroin) linctus (*Linctus diamorphinae*), 2 to 8 ml. (30 to 120 minims).

Phenazocine ('Narphen') is an analgesic of value in relieving pain in biliary colic.

Codeine (*Codeina*), 10–60 mg ($\frac{1}{6}$ to 1 grain)

This is an alkaloid derived from opium, having little tendency to promote habit formation. It has mild analgesic and hypnotic properties and depresses the cough reflex. It may be used for the latter purpose in the form of a linctus:

Codeine linctus (*Linctus codeinae*), 5 ml.

It is also included in 'Veganin' tablets (*Tabella Codeinae composita*) for its analgesic and hypnotic effects.

Dihydrocodeine bitartrate ('DF118') is a preparation which has powerful analgesic with only mild hypnotic properties. Dose: 10–60 mg.

Cannabis (Indian hemp or *Cannabis satira*) D.D.A.

This is the basis of hashish, the smoking of which is one of the forms of drug addiction. It is rarely used for therapeutic purposes. The following is a description of its action (Cushny, 1918) which is included here as an illustration of the effects of certain substances of this type on the drug addict.

"Soon after its administration, the patient passes into a dreamy, semiconscious state, in which the judgement seems to be lost, while the imagination is untrammelled by its usual restraints. The dreams assume the vividness of visions, are of boundless extravagance, and, of course, vary with the character and pursuits of the individual. In the eastern races they seem generally to partake of an amorous nature. The 'true believer' sees the gardens of paradise and finds himself surrounded by troops of houris of unspeakable beauty, while the less imaginative European finds himself unaccountably happy and feels constrained to active movement, often of a purposeless and even absurd character. Ideas flash through the mind without apparent continuity, and all measurement of time and space is lost."

The principal active ingredient of cannabis is tetrahydrocannabinol (TCH). A higher concentration of THC is found in the flowers than in the leaves. Marihuana ("pot") is a mixture of cannabis leaves and blossoms. Hashish is the resin from the tips of the female blossoms.

THC stimulates serotonin excretion in the brain and also releases catecholamines into the blood. Effects produced include a sensation of "time-stretching", intensification of odours, sound and colours and stimulation of appetite. "Pot" smokers tend to eat voraciously and care little what they eat.

Probably depending on dosage, people may be relaxed or aggressive after smoking cannabis. The eyes are suffused ("pink eye") but the extremities are vasoconstricted, making the hands cold.

At present cannabis has no medical uses, but research may well reveal some.

It has been argued in non-medical quarters that "pot" is harmless. However, cannabis may be deliberately adulterated with other substances, including opium. It is true that the purity of cannabis could be controlled if its sale were legalized, but there is no guarantee that addicts would not "graduate" to more harmful drugs as they sought more "way-out" experiences. The use of the other drugs, not only the "harder" ones but also "soft" ones like barbiturates, may result in premature death from starvation, exposure, psychosis, hepatitis or septicaemia.

Hyoscine also acts as a hypnotic and sedative (see p. 170).

III PSYCHOTROPIC DRUGS

In most cases these do not cure but substantially alleviate psychiatric disorders by suppressing symptoms until the condition remits spontaneously. The patient may also require discussion of his problems with a psychiatrist or with others (e.g. in group therapy), alteration of his environment (housing, employment, etc.), and perhaps other therapy.

DRUGS USED TO RELIEVE ANXIETY
(TRANQUILLIZERS, ATARACTICS, ANXIOLYTIC AGENTS)

An anxiety state may be primary or secondary to depression or an organic illness. For acute anxiety (e.g. panic attacks) sedation with a barbiturate, e.g. sodium amytal 45 mg t.d.s., is usually the treatment of choice. Other agents are preferable for the treatment of chronic anxiety.

Tranquillizers include meprobamate ('Equanil'), and the diazepine derivatives, i.e. chlordiazepoxide ('Librium'), diazepam ('Valium'), oxazepam ('Serenid-D') and medazepam ('Nobrium').

They are used in primary anxiety states and sometimes a single dose at night of meprobamate 400–800 mg or diazepam 10–15 mg will enable an obsessional anxious patient to fall asleep when ordinary hypnotics have failed.

Apart from their use in simple anxiety, diazepines are used to treat agitation in patients with depression and tension in patients with schizophrenia.

Phobic anxiety complicated by reactive depression often responds well to combined therapy with chlordiazepoxide and a monoamine oxidase inhibitor, e.g. phenelzine. Chlordiazepoxide in large doses is used in the treatment of alcohol and drug-withdrawal states.

The major tranquillizers (neuroleptics) are phenothiazines and butyrophenones, e.g. haloperidol ('Serenace'). Chlorpromazine ('Largactil'), promazine ('Sparine') and trifluoperazine ('Stelazine') are examples of phenothiazines and they are used for the treatment of schizophrenia, maniacal and confusional states. In schizophrenia they are taken for about two years after recovery. They can be combined with antidepressants to treat a depressed patient who is also tense and agitated. Phenothiazines are used in the treatment of a number of other conditions including vomiting, vertigo and pruritus. The dose of chlorpromazine is 25–100 mg orally or intramuscularly as a single dose or three or four times a day. Phenothiazines may cause extrapyramidal side-effects (e.g. abnormal movements and postures of the limbs) requiring prescription of an anti-Parkinsonian drug. They may also cause depression, jaundice, agranulocytosis and rashes.

Haloperidol is used for the control of over-activity, especially in mania. (1.5–6.0 mg b.d. orally, or 5–10 mg parenterally.

DRUGS USED TO TREAT DEPRESSION

Depression may be *reactive* (to environmental stress) or *endogenous* (without obvious external cause). Amphetamines are now obsolete in the treatment of depression, and the commonly used antidepressant drugs fall into two groups.

1. The mono-amine oxidase (MAO) inhibitors

Monoamine oxidase is an enzyme which destroys serotonin, adrenaline and noradrenaline. Depression may sometimes be caused by a deficiency of serotonin + noradrenaline in the brain. Some drugs inhibit the enzyme which destroys these hormones. Such drugs are called MAO inhibitors and examples are:

Iproniazid ('Marsilid')   Phenelzine ('Nardil')
Isocarboxazid ('Marplan')   Phenoxypropazine ('Drazine')
Mebanazine ('Actomol')   Tranylcypromine ('Parnate')
Nialamide ('Niamid')

If the patient is also anxious, chlordiazepoxide may be given at the same time.

Warning: Dangerous or even fatal idiosyncratic reactions to MAO inhibitors include jaundice and hypertensive crises, possibly causing a subarachnoid haemorrhage, when the patient eats foods containing tyramine, e.g. cheese, yoghourt, Bovril, Marmite and broad beans. Alcohol may also be dangerous. Ephedrine and amphetamines may similarly cause hypertensive crises and should not be administered to patients under treatment with MAO inhibitors. They should also be warned against taking 'Cold cures' which may contain phenylpropanolamine. Pethidine is also contraindicated in these patients, but for a different reason—it may cause hypotension, coma and convulsions.

2. The tricyclic antidepressants

Examples of these are:

Imipramine ('Tofranil')   Nortriptyline ('Aventyl')
Amitriptyline ('Tryptizol')   Trimipramine ('Surmontil')

The maintenance dose of all these is 50 mg t.d.s. Imipramine is useful when retardation (i.e. inertia) is prominent. The other three drugs have sedating effects and are used when agitation is prominent.

Protriptyline ('Concordin') and iprindole ('Prondol') act more rapidly than the above-mentioned drugs and have a more stimulating effect.

The side-effects of these drugs are a dry mouth, sweating, constipation and drowsiness.

Reactive depression responds better to a MAO inhibitor, and endogenous depression responds better to a tricyclic antidepressant.

Antidepressant drug therapy may take up to a fortnight to become effective, and if this time-lag is unacceptable (e.g. in severe depression) electroconvulsive therapy (E.C.T.) will be required. Antidepressant drugs potentiate one another and alarming reactions may occur if a MAO inhibitor is given together with a tricyclic antidepressant.

IV DRUGS WHICH STIMULATE THE NERVOUS SYSTEM

It has already been mentioned that certain drugs stimulate the respiratory and vasomotor centres in the medulla (e.g. nikethamide, leptazol, strychnine, caffeine). Strychnine and caffeine also have a stimulating effect on other parts of the nervous system and must be considered further. Cocaine also has a stimulating effect.

Caffeine (*Caffeina*), 300 mg (2 to 5 grains)

This drug has a number of actions:

1. Diuretic (p. 128).

2. Respiratory stimulant (p. 112).

3. Central nervous system stimulant. Caffeine excites the higher centres of the cerebrum, increasing mental activity and sensory impressions. It is often combined with aspirin and phenacetin (APC tablets).

Cocaine (*Cocaina*), 16 mg ($\frac{1}{8}$ to $\frac{1}{4}$ grain) D.D.A.

This drug has two important and opposite actions when used therapeutically. It stimulates the higher centres of the brain but depresses or paralyses the sensory endings of the peripheral nerves when applied locally (i.e. it acts as a local anaesthetic) (p. 158). The former action outweighs much of its value as a local anaesthetic and cocaine itself is only used occasionally. There are, however,

F

many substitutes specially prepared so that the effects on the higher centres are less marked.

Action on the higher centres. Cocaine stimulates the mental processes, producing hilarity and loquacity. In larger doses, it results in depression and finally coma. It is very prone to cause drug addiction and gives rise to serious results, with rapid mental and moral deterioration. For this reason its supply is most carefully guarded by the Dangerous Drugs Act.

Strychine (*Strychnina*), 2–8 mg ($\frac{1}{30}$ to $\frac{1}{8}$ grain)
    This is the alkaloid of nux vomica and was used as a constituent of some arrow poisons. The main points about its action are:
    1. The highest centres of the brain are not markedly affected by therapeutic doses, although possibly the senses do become more acute after its administration.
    2. It stimulates the spinal cord so that reflexes are increased and become brisker.
    3. Both strychnine and nux vomica are very bitter and act as "bitters" which improve the appetite and increase the tone of the stomach. They are used as "tonics".

    Strychnine poisoning. The main symptom is the occurrence of muscular spasms which, with larger doses, become generalized convulsions. They are due to stimulation of the spinal cord and resemble those occurring in tetanus. Consciousness remains unclouded.
    Treatment:
    (*a*) Gastric lavage.
    (*b*) Intravenous injection of thiopentone to control convulsions.
    (*c*) Barbiturate drugs by mouth.

Preparations of nux vomica and strychnine
    Tincture of nux vomica (*Tinctura nucis vomicae*), 2 ml. (10 to 30 minims).
    Strychnine mixture, B.P.C. Dose: 15 ml.
    Strychnine and iron mixture, B.P.C. Dose: 15 ml.

Amphetamine sulphate ('Benzedrine'), 2·5 to 10 mg ($\frac{1}{24}$ to $\frac{1}{6}$ grain)
    The following drugs have a similar action and uses:
        Dexamphetamine ('Dexedrine').
        Methyl amphetamine ('Methedrine').
    These synthetic drugs stimulate the higher centres, produce increased mental alertness and temporarily abolish fatigue. They are strongly habit-forming, i.e. addictive, and have been superseded by other drugs in the treatment of mental depression. Care should be taken not to give them near bed-time as they may result in insomnia. Locally they have an effect on the nasal mucous

membrane like adrenaline and ephedrine (i.e. they are vaso-constrictors) but are not now used for this purpose because of the danger of addiction. For the same reason, they are no longer recommended for the treatment of obesity.

Almost the only indication for amphetamines now is narcolepsy.

Methylphenidate ('Ritalin') is an alternative drug for the treatment of narcolepsy.

V ANTICONVULSANTS
(Epilepsy)

While it is not possible to state the cause of epilepsy it is clear that the seizures are associated with some local increase in the irritability of the cerebral cortex and that by reducing this irritability by means of anticonvulsant drugs which have a sedative action on the cortex, the fits are controlled or even abolished. The drugs used may be given either alone or two may be combined.

Phenobarbitone ('Luminal') 30–120 mg ($\frac{1}{2}$ to 2 grains) p. 130.

Methylphenobarbitone ('Prominal'). A drug similar in action to phenobarbitone which is said to produce less drowsiness and mental depression.

Phenytoin ('Epanutin', 'Solantoin', 'Dilantin', soluble phenytoin) 50–100 mg is used in some cases which do not respond well to phenobarbitone. Toxic symptoms often occur and include tremor, unsteadiness of movement, swelling of gums, rashes and indigestion. Occasionally megaloblastic anaemia occurs.

Sulthiame ('Ospolot'), 10–15 mg per kg body weight in divided doses.

Methoin ('Mesontoin'), 50–100 mg, $\frac{3}{4}$ to $1\frac{1}{2}$ grains.

Primidone ('Mysoline') 250–500 mg.

Phensuximide ('Milontin'), 1–3 G daily, and Ethosuximide ('Emeside', 'Zarontin') 250 to 1500 mg daily, are of value in *petit mal*.

Troxidone ('Tridione', 'Trimethadione'), 600 to 1800 mg daily in divided doses is sometimes employed in *petit mal*. Cases of agranulocytosis have followed its use which is, therefore, limited by its toxicity. 'Paradione' is also used for *petit mal*.

Bromides. The bromides of potassium, sodium or ammonium are occasionally used, 0·6–2 grams (10 to 30 grains).

For status epilepticus intramuscular injections of

(a) soluble phenobarbitone, 200 mg (3 grains) or

(b) paraldehyde, 5 ml. may be given.

VI DRUGS USED IN PARKINSONISM

Parkinsonism (e.g. paralysis agitans)

There are three particular facets of Parkinsonism which require treatment. They are:

(a) tremor

(b) rigidity

(c) hypokinesia (diminished mobility).

In general, drugs are more effective against rigidity than against tremor. Only L-dopa and amantidine relieve hypokinesia.

Antiparkinsonian drugs fall into several groups, viz.

1. Anticholinergic drugs, e.g. atropine, belladonna and stramonium.

Synthetic anticholinergic drugs are usually used and they include benzhexol ('Artane'), ethopropazine ('Lysivane'), orphenadrine hydrochloride ('Disipal'), procyclidine ('Kemadrin') and benztropine ('Cogentin').

2. Antihistamines

Drugs such as diphenhydramine ('Benadryl') and phenindamine ('Thephorin') may occasionally be of value.

3. L-dopa e.g. 'Larodopa'

This compound repletes the depleted dopamine levels in the brains of patients with Parkinsonism. Results are often dramatic and sometimes spectacular; patients who have long been chair-bound may walk again. Improvement occurs early but does not usually reach its maximum for six weeks or more. The starting dose is usually 0·5 to 1 G daily and dosage is increased by steps of 0·5 to 1 G daily at intervals of 3–4 days until the optimum dosage level is reached. Too rapid an increase or too high a dosage is liable to cause side-effects. The average daily dose is 6 G and the usual maximum is 8 G. The drug is given in divided doses, three or four times a day. The principal side-effect, nausea, may be abolished or lessened by giving the drug with food. Other side-effects are vomiting, anorexia, hypotension, cardiac dysrhythmias, flushing, mental changes and involuntary movements. Reduction of dosage is often all that is needed to abolish these side-effects.

4. Amantidine ('Symmetrel')

This compound has similar therapeutic effects to L-dopa, to which, however, it is chemically unrelated. Side-effects (e.g.

nervousness, insomnia, dizziness and psychiatric symptoms) are minimal and no elaborate build-up of dosage is necessary. The dose is 100 mg once daily for a week and thereafter 100 mg twice daily.

Either L-dopa or amantidine can be used in combination with other antiparkinsonian drugs and usually is.

VII DRUGS USED IN MIGRAINE

The patient may experience relief from mild analgesics such as aspirin, paracetamol or 'Veganin'. Other patients require **ergotamine**. This acts by constricting the painfully dilated extracranial arteries. It constricts other arteries at the same time and is therefore contraindicated in patients with serious vascular disease, e.g. coronary disease and hypertension. It is also contraindicated in pregnancy, because it stimulates the uterus to contract.

Ergotamine, to be effective, must be given very early in the attack. The most effective mode of administration is by subcutaneous or intramuscular injection (e.g. 'Femergin') 0·25–0·5 mg. Suppositories (2–6 mg) act quickly for patients who overcome the aesthetic objection to using them. Sublingual administration (e.g. 'Lingraine') 2 mg, or inhalation of a measured dose (0·36 mg) from an aerosol (e.g. 'Medihaler-Ergotamine') is, however, usually adequate and is certainly more convenient. Oral administration, of tablets to be swallowed, is the least effective but is adequate for some patients. The dose is 1–2 mg ergotamine, repeated half-hourly (to a maximum of 6 mg) until relief is obtained. Caffeine is often used to enhance the action of ergotamine, as in 'Cafergot' tablets and suppositories. In addition, in 'Migril' tablets, cyclizine is used to counteract nausea and vomiting due either to the disease or the ergotamine.

Phenobarbitone may reduce the frequency of attacks of migraine. Prochlorperazine ('Stemetil') and clonidine ('Catapres') are also used for this purpose, but is more toxic. Methysergide ('Deseril') is sometimes used when other drugs have failed. Its use is limited by occasional serious adverse reactions, e.g. retroperitoneal fibrosis which obstructs the ureters and causes hydronephrosis.

VIII DRUGS USED IN SOME OTHER CONDITIONS

Subacute combined degeneration of the cord. Vitamin B_{12} is necessary (p. 99).

Myasthenia gravis. Neostigmine (p. 168), piridostigmine and distigmine.

Trigeminal neuralgia. Carbamazepine ('Tegretol'), 200 mg, 6 hourly.

Chorea. Aspirin or sodium salicylate are given.

Syphilis of the nervous system. The usual antisyphilitic measures are employed.

Meningitis. Sulphonamide drugs are used for meningococcal, streptococcal and pneumococcal types (p. 228). In the latter two, penicillin is used simultaneously. Meningitis due to *Haemophilus influenzae* is treated with chloramphenicol and sulphadiazine.

Toxic substances acting on nerves

Lead, arsenic, mercury and alcohol may all have an action on the peripheral nerves resulting in peripheral neuritis. Various forms of paralysis ensue. The toxins of the diphtheria bacillus also have a special affinity for nervous tissue.

Local Anaesthetics (See also page 181)

I LOCAL (TOPICAL) APPLICATIONS TO MUCOUS MEMBRANES

Because of the thinness of the epithelium of mucous membranes, some drugs are absorbed and can easily reach and paralyse the sensory nerve endings in the vicinity.

(a) **Cocaine,** which is used as a solution (5 to 10 per cent) or ointment (4 to 10 per cent), especially in operations on the nose. The dangers of excessive absorption with toxic symptoms must always be remembered when cocaine is being used. (See also p. 153). Cocaine drops (2 per cent) are of value in anaesthetizing the conjunctiva prior to the removal of foreign bodies and eye operations. It also dilates the pupil. Amethocaine eye drops are usually preferable because they neither dilate the pupil nor damage the corneal epithelium which cocaine does. Solutions of these strengths must never be injected.

(b) **Amethocaine** ('Decicain', 'Pantocaine'), 1 to 2 per cent. This may be used in the same way as cocaine. It is also employed as a spray to anaesthetize the pharynx and larynx before the passage of a gastroscope and prior to bronchoscopy. It is less toxic than cocaine and, therefore, safer to use but is considerably more toxic than procaine.

(c) **Benzocaine** ('Anaesthesin') has a similar action and is employed as a lozenge or ointment. It is useful for painful or irritating lesions of the mouth and anus, viz:

Trochisci benzocainae compositi.
Unguentum benzocainae compositum.

II DRUGS GIVEN BY INJECTION (See also page 181)

These may be injected locally into the operation area (infiltration) or in the vicinity of the nerves which supply the area at some distance from the site of the operation (nerveblock). They should not be injected into inflamed or infected tissue. The most important are:

Lignocaine ('Xylocaine') is a local anaesthetic of low toxicity injected in strengths up to 2 per cent. It is a very stable substance, rapid in action which can be stored indefinitely and repeatedly sterilized in an autoclave. The maximum dose is 200 mg or 500 mg with adrenaline. It may be used as a topical application to mucous membranes (2 to 4 per cent solution). An ointment (5 per cent) is also available.

It is interesting to note that lignocaine may be used intravenously in the treatment of some disorders of cardiac rhythm, especially those following myocardial infarction.

Procaine ('Novocain' or 'Planocaine'). A solution having a strength of $\frac{1}{2}$ to 2 per cent is generally employed. It is occasionally given intravenously for special purposes (0·1% solution) but always without adrenaline.

Cinchocaine ('Nupercaine') formerly known as 'Percaine', which is also used as a spinal anaesthetic, must not be confused with procaine. It may be used locally but is very much stronger and more toxic than procaine and, therefore, weaker solutions are employed. It is also made in the form of an ointment.

Adrenaline (0·5 ml. of 1 in 1000 solution). This is often added to injected local anaesthetics in a dose not exceeding 0·5 mg or a greater concentration than 1 in 200,000. It should not be used when a digit is being anaesthetized. It acts on the blood vesels in the vicinity of the injection and constricts them, thereby diminishing the amount of local anaesthetic which can be carried away in the blood stream so that the duration of the anaesthesia is prolonged. In addition, the amount of bleeding is diminished.

III FREEZING THE SKIN

Ethyl chloride spray is sometimes employed and, by its rapid evaporation, freezes the area to which it is applied. The duration of the effect is very short and it is only suitable for incising superficial abscesses. Complete anaesthesia is not always obtained and the process of thawing may be painful.

A *most important warning* must be given in connection with the use of all local and spinal anaesthetics. The names of the substances employed are often similar and may be confused. Further, they are used in strengths varying from 0·5 per cent to 10 per cent. Fatal accidents have occurred from the substitution of 'Percaine' for procaine (hence the advantage of the name 'Nupercaine', or better still, cinchocaine for the former). Also mistakes can be made in reading the strengths on the labels by not observing the exact position of the decimal point. The nurse must therefore be most careful in handling these drugs and be quite sure that the one she is putting out for use is the correct one and in the strength in which it is ordered.

SPINAL ANAESTHESIA

1·5% lignocaine is introduced by means of lumbar puncture into the epidural (extradural) space of the spinal canal, where it surrounds the nerve roots in the neighbourhood of the injection. Here it paralyses the nervous tissue in the nerve roots so that impulses, both sensory and motor, are unable to pass. It follows that the motor impulses will not be able to pass from the anterior horn cells via the anterior nerve roots to the muscles which are, therefore, paralysed and completely relaxed. Likewise, sensory impulses coming from the periphery will not be able to enter the cord via the posterior nerve roots and pass up the sensory tracts to the brain. Therefore pain is not felt.

The paralysis also involves the nerves to the blood vessels of the limbs and abdominal organs which dilate and so accommodate more blood. There is thus less blood in the general circulation and the blood pressure tends to fall.

One of the most serious consequences of a fall in blood pressure is lack of blood to the brain. Lowering of the head of the operating table, an appropriate time after the spinal anaesthetic has been given, counteracts this effect of a fall in blood pressure.

If there are any signs of collapse during the operation, the head should be lowered in order to increase the blood supply to the brain, and a pressor drug such as metaraminol injected.

Epidural injection has superseded subarachnoid injection because it is safer.

CHAPTER 12

Drugs Acting on the Involuntary Nervous System

It will be recalled that the involuntary nervous system consists of the sympathetic system together with the cranial and sacral autonomic systems (parasympathetic), viz.:

Sympathetic system supplies
{
Pupils
Heart
Lungs, trachea, bronchi
Stomach and intestines
Suprarenal glands
Bladder
Uterus
}

Cranial autonomic supplies
{
Pupils
Heart
Lungs, trachea, bronchi
Stomach
}

Sacral autonomic supplies
{
Rectum
Bladder
Uterus
}

The nerve fibres pass mainly to involuntary, unstriped muscle in the walls of the various organs and also to the muscle in the walls of the arteries, i.e. the autonomic system supplies the viscera as distinct from the central nervous system which supplies the skeletal muscles.

A number of organs have both sympathetic and parasympathetic nerve-supplies which have opposite actions. Thus, the parasympathetic fibres which reach the heart carry impulses which slow the heart rate (inhibitors), while those from the sympathetic increase its rate (accelerators). The normal rate of the heart is maintained by a balance between the opposing impulses.

Further, the involuntary system is greaty influenced by the activities of the ductless glands. In particular the secretion from the suprarenal gland, adrenaline, stimulates the sympathetic system and acts as a vasoconstrictor.

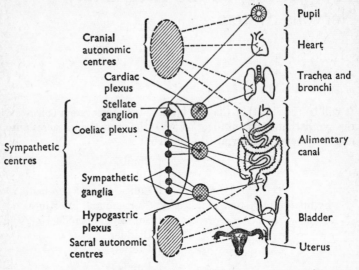

Fig. 5.—Illustrating distribution of involuntary nervous system.

Just as reflex action in the central nervous system takes place in the spinal cord, which receives afferent impulses and sends out efferent impulses, so reflex action occurs in the autonomic system through collections of nerve cells called ganglia. These ganglia also have connections with the spinal cord and brain. The sympathetic ganglia are situated in chains on either side of the vertebral column. The parasympathetic ganglia tend to be in or near the organ which they supply and are mainly grouped in the cranial and sacral autonomic centres.

Physiology. When an autonomic nerve is stimulated chemical substances are liberated which transmit the impulse at the nerve endings in the organ concerned. Other substances are also formed at the same time which antagonize the action of these stimulators and so prevent their effect being too powerful or too prolonged. These various substances differ in the sympathetic and parasympathetic nerve endings.

Parasympathetic stimulation liberates acetylcholine at the nerve endings. This is antagonized by cholinesterase.

Sympathetic stimulation liberates noradrenaline and adrenaline in addition to acetylcholine. At the same time adrenaline and noradrenaline may be secreted from the suprarenal glands. Monoamine oxidase (M.A.O.) antagonizes their action.

The involuntary system is somewhat complicated and classification of the drugs which affect it is made more difficult by the fact that they all differ in their mode of action. As a matter of convenience they may be divided into four main groups:

1. Those which produce results similar to stimulation of the sympathetic (sympathomimetic).

2. Those which "block" the action of adrenaline and noradrenaline on the sympathetic receptors in the tissues.

3. Those which produce results similar to stimulation of the parasympathetic (parasympathomimetic).

TABLE 4.—SUMMARY OF DRUG ACTION.

Organ	Effect of sympathetic stimulation (adrenaline)	Effect of parasympathetic stimulation (carbachol pilocarpine: eserine)	Action of Atropine
Pupils	Dilated	Contracted	Dilated
Heart rate	Increased	Decreased	Increased
Bronchial muscle	Relaxed	Contracted	Relaxed
Stomach movements and secretion	Decreased	Increased	Decreased
Saliva	Slight increase	Increased	Decreased
Bladder muscle	Relaxed	Contracted	Relaxed
Bladder sphincter	Contracted	Relaxed	Nil
Blood vessels	Contracted	Nil	Nil

4. The drugs of the atropine group (acetylcholine inhibitors).

Drugs acting on the involuntary nervous system may do so in a number of ways. Among the most important are:

1. General stimulants.

2. Ganglion-blocking agents which prevent reflex action taking place.

3. Drugs suppressing the action of (a) Cholinesterase thus increasing the action of acetylcholine. Such drugs are called anticholinesterases, an example being neostigmine.

(b) Monoamine oxidase thus increasing the action of adrenaline and nora-drenaline. Such drugs are called MAO inhibitors and they are used in the treatment of depression. An example is tranylcypromine ('Parnate').

Cheese contains tyramine which is normally destroyed by monoamine oxidase in the gut wall and liver and so causes no harm. MAO inhibitors allow the tyramine to enter the general circulation and to cause the release of noradrenaline from local stores. This results in acute severe hypertension which may cause a subarachnoid haemorrhage.

4. Drugs inhibiting the action of acetylcholine.

DRUGS ACTING AS SYMPATHETIC STIMULANTS

Adrenaline

Adrenaline or epinephrine is the active principle extracted from the medulla of the suprarenal glands, and, therefore, normally small amounts are continually passing from the glands into the blood stream. It is produced synthetically for therapeutic purposes.

If it is remembered that adrenaline stimulates the sympathetic system and that the symptoms of sympathetic stimulation are those which occur in fight or fright, i.e. those actions which are most necessary to the individual for self-preservation, it will not be difficult to understand some of its actions. Thus:

1. The maximum amount of blood is required for the muscles of the body, therefore there is a vasoconstriction of the blood vessels in the skin and alimentary organs. This also leads to a rise in blood pressure.

2. Glucose is needed in order to supply energy to the muscles, and so the liver liberates its store of glycogen into the blood.

3. The plain muscle of the bronchi is relaxed, thus allowing the maximum amount of air to enter the lungs.

Uses. (i) Relaxation of the spasm of the bronchial muscles in asthma (p. 118). Small doses of adrenaline 0·05 to 0·5 ml. of a 1 in 1000 solution, which is the strength in which adrenaline is generally used) are injected immediately the attack starts and are more efficacious than larger ones given when it is fully established. If the responsibility of administering the drug is left to the nurse, she should, therefore, give it as soon as possible. It is not uncommon to be summoned to a patient who has had an attack of asthma which has been in progress for a considerable period, for whom an injection of adrenaline has been ordered "p.r.n." and which could have been given by the nurse at its onset. An intelligent patient may be taught to give the injection to himself.

(ii) As a cardiac stimulant. By stimulating the heart and constricting the peripheral arteries and those of the abdominal organs the blood pressure is raised, so that adrenaline is sometimes used in the treatment of shock and collapse. The injection of adrenaline directly into the heart muscle will sometimes re-start the heart beating when it has stopped (cardiac arrest e.g. anaesthesia, asphyxia, drowning or carbon monoxide poisoning).

(iii) Adrenaline has a powerful local action in constricting the blood vessels when injected or applied to an open surface, i.e. it is a local haemostatic. Thus, it may be used as a spray or on gauze soaked in the solution for epistaxis, and for plugging a bleeding tooth socket (p. 55). Its value in delaying the absorption and so prolonging the action of a local anaesthetic has also been mentioned (p. 159).

(iv) It is sometimes used in allergic conditions such as urticaria and angio-neurotic oedema, and in anaphylaxis.

Adrenaline is destroyed by the digestive juices and so is inactive when given by mouth.

Preparations

Injection of adrenaline tartrate (*injectio adrenalini*, B.P.) is issued in ampoules of 0·5 ml. and 1·0 ml. The dose is 0·05 to 0·5 ml. subcutaneously, depending on age. Doses of 1 ml. are, however, sometimes given.

Solution of adrenaline hydrochloride (*Liquor adrenalinae hydrochloridi*, 1 in 1000), is not given by injection.

Other preparations include sprays, ointments and suppositories (in which it is sometimes combined with cocaine).

Isoprenaline (5–20 mg) has a similar action to adrenaline and may be given either by inhalation or in the form of tablets which are allowed to dissolve under the tongue. It is frequently used in the treatment of asthma. 'Saventrine', a long-acting form of isoprenaline, is of value in the treatment of chronic heart block.

Noradrenaline (dose 2 to 8 micrograms per minute by intravenous infusion) is a hormone secreted by sympathetic nerve endings and by the adrenal medulla, also produced synthetically, which raises blood pressure by acting as a vasoconstrictor. It is sometimes used in the treatment of shock and collapse (p. 90).

'Levophed' is a preparation which may be used.

(N.B.—One ampoule contains 4 ml. of 1 in 1000 solution. 1 ml. contains the equivalent of 1 mg of noradrenaline. One ampoule, 4 ml. is added to 1000 ml. of saline or dextrose which is infused at the rate of 0·5 to 2 ml. per minute by intravenous drip.)

Ephedrine (*Ephedrina*), 16–60 mg (¼ to 1 grain)

This is an alkaloid obtained from a Chinese plant, but can also be prepared by chemical means. Its action and uses are very similar to those of adrenaline. It is, however, slower and more prolonged in action and has advantages when used in some conditions. For example, it is given before a spinal anaesthetic because the rise in blood pressure is more prolonged than that obtained by adrenaline. Unlike adrenaline, it can be given by mouth and is employed in regular doses between attacks of asthma in order to reduce their frequency.

Ergotamine tartrate

This is an alkaloid which is extracted from ergot (a drug used for its effect on the uterus, p. 212). Although it has some actions which are similar to those of adrenaline, it is not used for the same purpose but may be conveniently mentioned here. Its most important action is to constrict the blood vessels (vasoconstriction). This may be so marked that if used in excessive doses or over a long period it may lead to gangrene of the extremities. It is sometimes used in the treatment of migraine (p. 157).

It may be given (*a*) by injection (0.25 to 0.5 milligram), (*b*) by mouth (1 to 4 milligrams), when tablets should be placed under the tongue. A proprietary preparation is known as 'Femergin'.

SYMPATHETIC (ADRENERGIC) RECEPTORS

The sympathetic nervous system exerts its effects via receptors which are present in various tissues. The receptors are of two kinds—alpha (α) and beta (β). The α-receptors are *excitatory* and the α-receptors are generally *inhibitory:* an important exception is in the heart, where the β-receptors are excitatory.

Stimulation of α-receptors causes contraction of smooth muscle in the walls of blood vessels, and hence *vasoconstriction*, contraction of the iris, with consequent *dilation of the pupil*, contraction of the sphincter of the urinary bladder and contraction of the pilomotor muscles—the little muscles which make hairs stand up. One substance which stimulates α-receptors is **noradrenaline.** The action of noradrenaline is inhibited by drugs, such as phentolamine ('Rogitine'), which block the α-receptors.

Stimulation of the β-receptors results in relaxation of smooth muscle in the walls of blood vessels, and hence *vasodilatation*, especially in skeletal muscles, relaxation of smooth muscle in the walls of bronchi, with consequent *bronchodilatation*, relaxation of smooth muscle in the walls of the intestines, relaxation of the muscular wall of the urinary bladder and stimulation of the heart so that it beats more rapidly and more forcibly. **Isoprenaline** is a drug which stimulates β-receptors and thereby produces these effects. **Adrenaline** stimulates both α- and β-receptors, the result being the sum of all the effects mentioned. The effect of adrenaline on a tissue depends on the affinity of the substance for the receptors and on the proportions of the two types of receptor in the tissue. **Propranolol** is a β-receptor blocking agent and prevents the stimulation of β-receptors by noradrenaline or adrenaline. It is of value in cases of angina pectoris because it inhibits sympathomimetic influences and consequently slows the heart, reduces its force of contraction and decreases its oxygen consumption. It is also effective against certain disturbances of cardiac rhythm.

Propranolol is contraindicated in patients with asthma since it inhibits the bronchodilating effects of adrenaline and may result in bronchospasm. More recently introduced β-receptor blocking agents, e.g. practolol ('Eraldin') and oxprenolol ('Trasicor'), are more selective in their action on the heart and may be used in asthmatic patients.

DRUGS ACTING AS PARASYMPATHETIC STIMULANTS

There are a number of drugs which have an action similar to that of the parasympathetic system. Their main actions are:

1. To stimulate the muscular movements of the bowel, i.e. to increase peristalsis. They are therefore used in conditions in which the gut is distended, e.g. postoperative distension, paralytic ileus, acute dilation of the stomach, certain types of constipation.

2. To dilate the blood vessels in the limbs in conditions such as Raynaud's disease. Their injection may, therefore, be associated with a fall in blood pressure.

3. To relax the sphincter of the bladder, e.g. postoperative retention of urine.

Group I. Acetylcholine type

Mecholyl, 10 milligrams

Carbachol ('Doryl', 'Moryl'), 0·25 mg.

Group II. Anticholinesterase drugs

Physostigmine ('Eserine'), 0·6–1·2 mg ($\frac{1}{100}$ to $\frac{1}{50}$ grain)

This is an alkaloid which has two main uses:

(i) To relieve paralytic conditions of the bowel, e.g. post-operative distension, but drugs such as carbachol have tended to replace it.

(ii) To contract the pupil of the eye, e.g. in the treatment of glaucoma (p. 215).

Neostigmine ('Prostigmin')

This is a similar drug used especially in the treatment of myasthenia gravis. It may also be used in paralytic ileus and atony of the bladder. The dose given by mouth is about 15 milligrams, or by injection, 1 milligram.

Pilocarpine (*Pilocarpina*), 3–12 mg ($\frac{1}{20}$ to $\frac{1}{5}$ grain).

This is an alkaloid obtained from a plant. It has two main actions:
(i) It stimulates the secretion of sweat and saliva (pp 55, 60).
(ii) It contracts the pupil of the eye.

Drugs inhibiting action of acetylcholine (atropine group)

Atropine (*Atropina*), 0·25–1 mg ($\frac{1}{240}$ to $\frac{1}{60}$ grain)

Atropine is an alkaloid obtained from the belladonna plant (Deadly Nightshade), and the effects of belladonna preparations in the body are mainly due to the atropine which they contain. Atropine has many actions and is used for a number of therapeutic purposes.

Action on plain muscle. Atropine relaxes plain muscle. Thus it helps to relax the spasm of the bronchial muscle in asthma. It relaxes spasm in the muscle of the bile duct and ureter and so is of value in the treatment of biliary and renal colic.

Action on secretions. Atropine diminishes the secretion of the salivary glands, the sweat glands and the glands in the mucous membrane of the respiratory tract.

Its power of diminishing the secretion of mucus from the respiratory tract is made use of in the pre-anaesthetic injection of atropine. It is also employed in the treatment of pulmonary oedema and in some cases of bronchitis.

It may be given with morphine to prevent the accumulation of bronchial secretion in the lungs, because morphine depresses the cough reflex and if an excess of mucus is present it may accumulate in the smaller bronchioles.

Action on the stomach. Atropine diminishes the movements of the stomach and also the amount of gastric juice secreted. It is therefore sometimes used in the treatment of gastric ulcer in the acute stages. It also tends to diminish intestinal movements and spasms and so may be given in cases of colic.

Action on the eye (p. 214). Atropine when given by hypodermic injection or instilled into the conjunctival sac, dilates the pupils. Atropine drops are therefore employed to dilate the pupils in cases of iritis, eye injury and for purposes of examination.

Action on the heart. Atropine blocks the inhibitory effect of the vagus nerve and so causes an increase in heart rate and contractility. This action is of value when bradycardia and hypotension complicate acute myocardial infarction.

Poisoning. Poisoning by atropine or belladonna produces the following symptons:

1. Dryness of the mouth and throat with hoarseness of the voice.

2. Wide dilation of the pupils.

3. Stimulation of the higher centres of the nervous system which is not apparent when therapeutic doses are used, viz. restlessness, talkativeness, delirium and often violent maniacal excitement. With large doses this stage of excitement soon passes off and is followed by depression developing into coma.

4. Skin eruptions, e.g. generalized erythema, may be present.

Treatment

1. Gastric lavage.

2. Tannic acid, 1·2 gram (20 grains) in 115 ml. (4 ounces) of water, as an antidote to precipitate ingested atropine.

3. Artificial ventilation and oxygen.

4. Neostigmine two-hourly until skin becomes moist.

Preparation of belladonna

Tincture of belladonna (*Tinctura belladonnae*), 0·3 to 2 ml. (5 to 30 minims).

For external application:

Glycerin of belladonna (*Glycerinum belladonnae*).

Belladonna plaster (*Emplastrum belladonnae*).

These preparations are applied externally for the relief of pain, and possibly act as counter-irritants.

Preparations of atropine

Atropine Sulphate Injection, B.P. 0·25 to 2 mg ($\frac{1}{240}$ to $\frac{1}{30}$ grain).
Atropine Sulphate Tablets, B.P. 0·25 to 2 mg ($\frac{1}{240}$ to $\frac{1}{30}$ grain).
Most of the other preparations, e.g. ointments and drops, are used for eye conditions (p. 214).

Substances like atropine

Homatropine (p. 214). Used in eye work to dilate the pupil.
Atropine methonitrate ('Eumydrin') (p. 66). Used in congenital pyloric stenosis and whooping cough.

Hyoscine hydrobromide (Scopolamine), 0·3–0·6 mg ($\frac{1}{200}$ to $\frac{1}{100}$ grain).

This is one of the alkaloids obtained from hyoscyamus. Some of its actions resemble those of atropine but it does not cause tachycardia. In addition, it depresses the central nervous system and so has an hypnotic action. It has the following uses:

1. As an hypnotic, by injection, in the treatment of mania and acute delirium, including delirium tremens, etc., although in some cases it appears to increase excitement.

2. To relieve the spasm and muscular rigidity in paralysis agitans. Like atropine, it inhibits the secretion of saliva and dryness of the mouth may be produced. This is counteracted by giving pilocarpine, 6 mg ($\frac{1}{10}$ grain), at the same time. In this instance hyoscine is given by mouth in the form of a tablet.

3. To prevent travel sickness.

Hyoscyamus

This is the dried leaf of a plant. It is mainly used for the treatment of bladder conditions. Preparations include a tincture (dose, 2–4 ml., 30–60 minims) and dry and liquid extracts.

Synthetic anticholinergic drugs, such as **propantheline** ('Probanthine') reduce secretion and motility in the gastrointestinal tract and are therefore used in the treatment of peptic ulcer.

CHAPTER 13

Drugs used in General Anaesthesia

Although chloroform, introduced by Simpson in 1847, was the first anaesthetic to come into general use, the anaesthetic properties of nitrous oxide were observed by Davy in 1788 and Long used ether in 1842. In more recent years many new substances have been discovered and employed in addition to those substances given by intravenous injection and the use of local, spinal and nerve-blocking injections. Chloroform, in particular, has largely fallen into disuse. The fact that it is non-inflammable has been an advantage when diathermy has been employed or when there has been a possibility of the development of static electricity in the operating theatre—a spark from which may ignite an explosive mixture.

GENERAL ANAESTHESIA

Drugs used in the production of general anaesthesia fall into three main classes:

1. Volatile substances the vapour of which is inhaled, e.g.

Chloroform	Trichlorethylene ('Trilene')
Ether	Divinyl ether ('Vinesthene')
Ethyl chloride	Halothane (Fluothane)

2. Gases such as:

Nitrous oxide	Cyclopropane

3. Substances given by:
   Intravenous injection, e.g. Thiopentone sodium ('Pentothal')
   Rectal injection, e.g. Bromethol ('Avertin')

Preoperative preparation
   (a) General.
   (b) Immediate (premedication).

(a) **General.** Most patients about to undergo an operation have some degree of apprehension. Therefore, reassurance reinforced, if necessary, by some sedative drug is usually required. Breathing exercises are desirable especially in patients with chronic chest disease and suitable antibiotics to control any infection may be necessary. Special conditions such as diabetes may need careful adjustment of diet and drugs; any anaemia should be corrected by blood transfusion before and during operation or treated with anti-anaemic drugs if time permits. Patients on steroids require special consideration and additional doses may be required. Patients being treated with the monoamine oxidase inhibitors (MAOI) e.g., iproniazid ('Marsilid'), phenelzine ('Nardil'), isocarboxazid ('Marplan'), tranylcypromine ('Parnate') should not receive pethidine as they greatly enhance its effect.

In other words, before anaesthesia an enquiry should always be made into the general health of the patient and any drugs which he may be taking.

(b) **Premedication before general anaesthesia.** (i) A barbiturate or other suitable sedative the night before operation is usually desirable.

(ii) Immediate premedication 1–1½ hours before with papaveretum ('Omnopon'), 10 to 20 mg, and hyoscine ('Scopolamine'), 0·2 to 0·4 mg, is usually employed. Atropine, which helps to dry secretions, may be used instead of hyoscine.

N.B.—Morphine and allied substances (papaveretum) should be used with the greatest caution, if ever, in young children. Atropine (0·2 to 0·4 mg/kg body weight may be all that is required; it may produce tachycardia but it is usually well tolerated by young children. Rectal thiopentone may be used as a preoperative sedative if it is desired to avoid injections.

Postoperative management

With the use of muscle relaxants modern anaesthetic techniques are generally directed to light anaesthesia. Restlessness and vomiting may therefore occur early and even during the transfer of the patient from the operating theatre to the bed. At all times one of the most important things is to keep a clear airway and to ensure that the tongue does not fall backwards, by pulling the tongue forwards with the finger if necessary and then turning the head or body to one side and holding the jaw forwards. If vomiting occurs the head should be lowered and a suction apparatus employed.

In many severe cases the patient is moved directly into a recovery ward or intensive care unit before return to a general ward. Intravenous drips, blood transfusion and oxygen administration must be continued as required. Solid food is generally withheld for 12–24 hours but sips of fluid are permitted when consciousness has returned.

Stages of anaesthesia

Basically there are three stages during the induction of general anaesthesia especially with ether but with modern premedication or the use of intravenous anaesthetics these are not usually observed.

Stage 1. Mental dullness and analgesia.

Stage 2. Excitement.

Stage 3. Surgical anaesthesia.

1. The stage of mental dullness. The first effect is a sensation of slight suffocation and warmth of the body due to dilation of the blood vessels in the skin. The senses become less acute, voices appear distant and may be replaced by ringing sounds and other noises. The patient has a "far away" feeling and to some extent the appreciation of pain becomes dulled though not necessarily abolished.

2. The stage of excitement. This is variable. In children it is often non-existent; in some, scarcely evident; in others, slight movements may become violent struggles, secrets may become common property, bad language in one person may have its counterpart in prayer in another, abuse may alternate with protestations of affection, while the vocal efforts may be ecclesiastical in character, operatic or reminiscent of the music hall.

3. The stage of anaesthesia. The third stage of complete anaesthesia is ushered in as the muscles relax and the struggles cease. Vocal refrains give place to regular breathing, which tends to become slower and more shallow as the depth of anaesthesia increases. The pupils contract somewhat, only to dilate again if the anaesthesia becomes dangerously deep, the corneal reflex is lost and finally there is no longer any pupillary reaction to light. The cough reflex is abolished and unless the jaw is supported, the tongue tends to fall back and impede respiration.

The pulse generally remains steady in rate and regular in rhythm, unless the patient is gravely ill or the operation is very prolonged, when it may become more rapid, weaker and, sometimes, irregular. Blood pressure tends to fall a little, except with ether anaesthesia, during which it is generally maintained. In some instances the fall may be considerable and cause grave anxiety.

During recovery, the patient returns to consciousness through the same stages, although they may be less obvious. Reflexes return, there is often some degree of restlessness and, finally, a period of drowsiness and dulled mental state before full recovery is attained.

Summary

(i) Anaesthetics given by inhalation reach the lungs in the inspired air. They pass through the alveoli into the blood, by which they are carried in the red corpuscles to the cells of the brain. Here they act by depressing the activity of the cells to such an extent that consciousness is lost.

(ii) The tendon, pupillary and corneal reflexes are lost.

(iii) The cough and vomiting reflexes are lost.

(iv) The muscles are relaxed.

(v) The blood pressure falls progressively with increasing depth of anaesthesia in the cases of chloroform, ether and halothane.

(vi) The blood vessels of the skin are dilated. Therefore, there is a tendency to considerable loss of heat from the body. This is minimized by clothing the patient suitably in a flannel gown and woollen stockings, by hot blankets and by maintaining the temperature of the operating theatre.

(vii) Volatile anaesthetics are excreted from the body mainly by the lungs. Therefore the inhalation of carbon dioxide and oxygen mixture after the administration has ceased stimulates the respiratory centre so that the increased rate and depth of breathing hastens their excretion (p. 113).

N.B.—There are three important questions which a nurse should ask, and verify, of every patient about to have a general anaesthetic,

1. Have you any false teeth?
2. Have you had any food or drink during the last four hours?
3. Is the bladder empty?

Chloroform

This is a heavy volatile liquid having a characteristic sweetish odour and is a very powerful anaesthetic. Its only advantage is that it is non-inflammable and non-explosive. On the other hand, it is very dangerous because it causes severe depression of the vaso-motor centre and myocardial depression with cardiac arrest. In the presence of adrenaline it may lead to ventricular fibrillation and may later have a fatal toxic effect on the liver (delayed chloroform poisoning.) Therefore, it is now rarely, if ever, used.

Ether (diethyl ether)

This is a light, colourless, highly volatile liquid which evaporates very quickly and produces a marked cooling of the body surface to which it is applied. It dissolves fat and oil and is sometimes used for cleaning the skin, especially when an injured area is contaminated with oil or grease. It undergoes chemical change if exposed to strong light and is therefore kept in amber-coloured bottles.

It may be administered by the "open method" on a mask or by a "closed method" using a special anaesthetic apparatus. The endotracheal (intratracheal) route may also be used.

It has the following advantages as an anaesthetic:

(i) It does not depress the respiratory centre or the heart except in large doses and, therefore, there is a considerable margin of safety in its administration. Chloroform is twenty-five times more toxic to the heart.

(ii) It does not tend seriously to lower the blood pressure and so is useful in cases of shock.

Disadvantages include:

(i) It tends to irritate the bronchial mucous membrane.

(ii) It is highly inflammable and, when mixed with air or oxygen forms a highly explosive mixture. Under no circumstances must there be a naked light or any apparatus liable to produce a spark, e.g. diathermy; or high temperature, e.g. the electric cautery, in the room while ether is being used.

Metal anaesthetic trolleys and operating tables, etc., with rubber castors are liable to carry a charge of electricity which may produce a small spark, and this has been sufficient to cause explosions and fires, having fatal results. It is therefore customary to "earth" such apparatus by means of a metal chain which makes contact with the ground and to use trolleys with special wheels. "Anti-static" wheels are coloured yellow.

Ethyl chloride

This is a very volatile liquid which evaporates so rapidly that it produces a freezing effect on the skin. Advantage is taken of this to produce local anaesthesia. It has an unpleasant smell and, for purposes of general anaesthesia, is often mixed with eau de Cologne. Ethyl chloride has a powerful action and induces anaesthesia rapidly. It is only suitable for short operations lasting a few minutes, e.g. incision of abscesses, etc., and for inducing anaesthesia which is continued by the administration of ether.

It is usually given on an open mask.

Trichlorethylene ('Trilene')

This is a useful, non-inflammable anaesthetic which is less toxic than chloroform. It is non-irritant to the respiratory passages but does not produce the complete muscular relaxation necessary for some major operations. It may be used in obstetrics. An added blue colour distinguishes it from other liquids.

Divinyl ether ('Vinesthene')

This is a volatile liquid with a very potent anaesthetic vapour. It is used for rapid induction of anaesthesia, particularly in children.

Halothane ('Fluothane')

The vapour of this volatile liquid is a potent anaesthetic. It causes a fall in blood pressure, which may be undesirable. Very rarely, hepatitis has occurred after operations performed under halothane anaesthesia and is probably due to an immunological reaction.

II. GASEOUS SUBSTANCES

Nitrous oxide (N_2O)

Nitrous oxide is a colourless gas having a very faint odour and sweetish taste. It is the oldest anaesthetic and its early name "laughing gas" is indicative of the hilarity which may be produced during the excitement stage of induction or recovery. It is stored in cylinders and administered via a bag and rubber face-piece, either directly from the cylinders for short anaesthesia, or by means of more elaborate apparatus for prolonged administration. Advantages:

(i) It is a very safe anaesthetic if administered with 20 to 40% oxygen.

(ii) It does not lower blood pressure or increase shock.

(iii) It rarely produces vomiting.

(iv) It may be given by the endotracheal method or nasally.

Disadvantages:

(i) Cumbersome and expensive apparatus is necessary for its administration.

(ii) It is not always possible to obtain full muscular relaxation without adequate premedication with a hypnotic or basal anaesthetic, and the addition of ether may be necessary. The quantity of ether required, however, is much less than when ether is used alone and, in this respect, nitrous oxide is one of the most useful anaesthetics available.

Use in midwifery. Inhalations of nitrous oxide and oxygen are supplied pre-mixed (50 per cent of each) in a cylinder and administered by the patient herself with an Entonox apparatus.

Cyclopropane

This is a non-irritating gas which has powerful anaesthetic properties. It can be given with large amounts of oxygen, with which it may form an explosive mixture. It is only used with safety by experts, but has advantages which render it especially valuable in thoracic surgery.

III. SUBSTANCES GIVEN BY INJECTION

A. Substances given by intravenous injection

(a) Barbiturates

(i) As general anaesthetics for short operations.

(ii) For longer operations if repeated doses are given or a continuous drip method employed.

(iii) For induction of anaesthesia followed by ether or nitrous oxide.

(iv) As basal anaesthetics.

(v) To control the spasms of tetanus.

They are all extremely quick in action, the patient passing into unconsciousness in less than 30 seconds if given rapidly. The effect of a full single dose of 'Pentothal' lasts about 15 minutes; that of 'Brietal' for 5 to 7 minutes. This may be prolonged, as stated above, by repeated injections of smaller doses or by a continuous drip method.

Great care must be taken to maintain an efficient airway. The jaw, which always tends to fall back even before the injection has been completed, must be properly supported until recovery from the anaesthetic is in sight.

The patient must be lying flat during the administration as a fall in blood pressure is produced and, if the patient were allowed to sit up, e.g. in a dental chair, the lack of blood supply to the brain might be sufficient to produce dangerous symptoms. Twitching of the muscles, which may be violent, is sometimes observed.

The solutions are strong irritants and it is most important that none should get into the tissues surrounding the vein.

The immediate injection of 'Hyalase' in normal saline into the area is helpful.

Accidental injection into an artery is even more serious and may lead to gangrene. It is treated by immediate injection of 10 ml. of 1% procaine into the artery.

Thiopentone sodium, B.P. ('Pentothal')

0·25–0·5 gram is dissolved in 10 ml. of sterile distilled water before injection. About 5 to 10 ml. are generally required to induce anaesthesia.

Methohexital sodium ('Brietal sodium')

50–120 mg intravenously, gives a short period of anaesthesia with quick, recovery. It is also useful for induction of more prolonged anaesthesia.

(b) Eugenol derivatives e.g. propanidid

This group of drugs is derived from oil of cloves. Their action is brief and they are useful in cases where an extremely rapid recovery of consciousness is required. Unlike barbiturates they do not cause a hangover and they are therefore useful for minor operations on out-patients. Propanidid is, however, more likely than barbiturates to cause postoperative vomiting and this is a definite drawback to use of the drug.

Measures which may be adopted in an emergency during general anaesthesia include:

Artificial respiration and external cardiac massage.

Inhalation of oxygen.

Cardiac massage after opening the thorax.

B. Substances given by rectal injection

These are not now often used as "basal anaesthetics" with the object of rendering the patient drowsy or unconscious before reaching the operating theatre. Their disadvantages are that respiration may be depressed and that once the dose has been given and absorbed it is slowly excreted so that should the patient collapse little can be done to hasten the recovery from the anaesthetic. They include:

Bromethol ('Avertin')

This still has a use in the treatment of some cases of eclampsia but may be definitely contraindicated in some associated diseases.

The patient must be closely supervised by a nurse from the time bromethol is given until consciousness is regained.

Paraldehyde

This drug, which is described under hypnotics (p. 141), is sometimes given in appropriate doses per rectum as a basal anaesthetic. Up to 4 ml. (60 minims) per stone body weight is given in saline to make a 10 per cent solution. It is less powerful than bromethol.

AIDS TO ANAESTHESIA

Muscle relaxants

1. Tubocurarine. Preparations of curare and similar substances, e.g. 'Tubarine', gallamine triethiodide ('Flaxedil'), are given by injection in order to increase muscular relaxation, thus diminishing the amount of general anaesthetic necessary. These drugs act by competing with acetylcholine, the normal chemical transmitter, at the neuromuscular junction. A test dose of 5 mg of tubocurarine is often given intravenously to detect unusually sensitive individuals. If after four minutes there is no indication of unusual sensitivity, another 10 to 25 mg are given. Repeated doses are given as necessary during the course of the operation. If recovery of respiration is delayed after tubocurarine, its action can be antagonized with neostigmine, 1 to 5 mg intravenously, preceded by atropine 1 mg.

Apart from its use in anaesthesia, tubocurarine may be used in the treatment of tetanus and in a diagnostic test for myasthenia gravis.

2. Suxamethonium ('Scoline'). The usual dose is 25 to 100 mg intravenously. Suxamethonium produces neuromuscular block by depolarizing the motor end plates in muscle. It rapidly produces profound muscular relaxation of brief duration (less than 5 minutes). It facilitates endotracheal intubation and is also useful in electroconvulsive therapy (ECT). There is no specific antagonist to suxamethonium. Neostigmine prolongs its action. Normal individuals possess an enzyme (cholinesterase) which destroys suxamethonium. Some individuals exist who have a hereditary abnormality or deficiency of the enzyme and cannot therefore destroy the drug. These patients fail to resume spontaneous breathing after suxamethonium administration. They have to be maintained on a mechanical ventilator until the relaxant has been excreted or until sufficient cholinesterase has been given by way of fresh blood transfusion.

3. Mephenesin ('Myanesin'), 0·5–1 gram (30–15 ml. of 2% solution by slow intravenous injection). This is a synthetic substance which produces some muscular relaxation, but generally insufficient for surgery. It appears to act on the spinal cord and may be used in strychnine poisoning and tetanus.

It is also used as a general muscle relaxant in a nunber of spastic conditions and may be given by mouth in the form of an elixir or 0·5 G tablets. It may be used in sedative preparations given in anxiety states.

Induced hypotension

Reducing the blood pressure will diminish bleeding during an operation which may thereby be conducted in a relatively bloodless field. This may be important when fine structures may have to be identified, as in neurosurgery and E.N.T. surgery. There are various means of inducing a controlled fall in blood pressure and the easiest is to administer hypotensive drugs, usually ganglion-blocking agents, intravenously. Postoperatively the patient must be left lying supine unless express orders are given to the contrary. If the patient is sat up before the effect of the drug has fully worn off, his blood pressure may drop dangerously. Suitable ganglion-blockers are trimetaphan ('Arfonad') and phenactropinium ('Trophenium'), both of which are short-acting and are usually given as a continuous intravenous infusion.

Halothane by itself may produce a surgically-adequate degree of hypotension and ganglion-blockers are used less frequently than they were.

Vasopressors have little place in anaesthesia but it is important to know about them. In shock the emphasis is on restoring the blood volume with suitable intravenous fluids, usually blood or dextran preparations. Hypotension due to adrenal insufficiency is treated with hydrocortisone intravenously.

Vasopressors which may be used include methoxamine ('Vasoxine') 2 mg intravenously, metaraminol ('Aramine') 2–10 mg intramuscularly or intravenously, or, as a last resort, noradrenaline ('Levophed'). Adrenaline or adrenaline-like drugs, such as metaraminol (sympathomimetic amines), must not be administered to patients receiving chloroform, cyclopropane or trichlorethylene, as dangerous disorders of cardiac rhythm and even ventricular fibrillation may result. Methoxamine is particularly useful in anaesthesia because it is compatible with cyclopropane and halothane. Any vasopressor must be used only with the greatest of caution in patients with cardiovascular disease or thyrotoxicosis.

Hypothermia

In some operations it may be necessary or desirable to stop or restrict the blood flow to the heart or brain (or other organs). Neither organ could normally tolerate this for long because each has a great need for oxygen which, of course, is carried in the blood.

The need for oxygen is, however, governed by the metabolic rate which may be reduced by cooling the patient. This gives more time, although for many cardiac operations it is not enough and a pump-oxygenator (heart–lung machine) is necessary.

Cooling may be achieved by immersing the body in cold water, or by passing the blood through a heat exchanger. Whichever method is adopted, drugs may be used to facilitate cooling. These drugs prevent shivering which would increase oxygen consumpton and would also retard the process of cooling. Chlorpromazine (given as a premedication) acts centrally to abolish shivering and the vasoconstrictor response to cold, and acts peripherally as a vaso-dilator, both of which actions facilitate cooling. Muscular relaxants and also anaesthetics themselves prevent shivering, and the latter have a vasodilator effect which increases heat loss from the skin.

LOCAL ANAESTHETICS (See also page 158)

Local anaesthetics are drugs which paralyse the sensory nerves in the region of their application, so that the passage of painful stimuli towards the spinal cord becomes impossible. Motor nerves in the vicinity are also affected. They may be used in the following ways:

1. Direct local applications to mucous membranes, e.g. cocaine.

2. By injection, the same drugs being used for all the following:

(*a*) Injection into the skin and tissues at the site of the operation.

(*b*) Injection around nerves at some distance from the site of the operation so that the area which they supply is anaesthetized, i.e. "regional anaesthesia" produced by nerve-block.

(*c*) "Splanchnic nerve-block", i.e. injection of the nerve ganglia on the posterior abdominal wall which receive the nervous impulses from the abdominal viscera such as the stomach and gall bladder. This is combined with local anaesthesia of the abdominal wall for some operations.

3. Freezing the skin with ethyl chloride spray.

The ideal requirements of a local anaesthetic are:

1. To paralyse the sensory nerves without damaging them or the surrounding tissues.

2. To be easily sterilized.

3. To be devoid of toxic effects after absorption.

4. To produce anaesthesia of sufficient duration for the operation to be performed and to leave no after-effects.

CHAPTER 14

Vitamins and Drugs used in Disorders of Metabolism

THE VITAMINS

Vitamins or accessory food factors are substances the presence of which in the food is essential for normal health and growth.

They are found in many natural foodstuffs but, in order to maintain health, only minute quantities, compared with the bulk of other articles of diet, are required.

Our knowledge of their composition and nature has increased rapidly in recent years and it is now possible to manufacture a number of them in the laboratory. In many instances it is these synthetic products which are used in therapeutics.

Deficiencies may be serious in underdeveloped countries and in times of war and famine. It should be made clear, however, that vitamin deficiency is rare in this country and that their addition to a normal diet is rarely necessary, except perhaps in the case of infants, nursing mothers, and elderly persons who may not look after themselves properly. In other words, quantities are prescribed and consumed unnecessarily and it must be remembered that prolonged overdosage (especially of vitamin D) may be dangerous.

But some special diets may be deficient in vitamins and in some diseases their absorption may not be adequate.

Vitamin A (Axerophthol)

Sources. This fat-soluble vitamin is found especially in milk, butter, egg-yolk, cod-liver oil, spinach, raw carrots and other vegetables. It is formed in the walls of the small intestine from carotene, a yellow pigment found in certain vegetables.

Effects. Its deficiency, which is rare, produces:

(i) A disorder of the eyes called xerophthalmia.

(ii) Night-blindness or difficulty experienced by some people in seeing in the dark.

(iii) Roughness and dryness of the skin resulting from changes in the epithelium which may lead to diminished resistance to infection both of the skin and mucous membranes.

Vitamin A is necessary for health and growth of the young.

Vitamin B

A number of separate substances having different actions are obtained from this group of water-soluble vitamins.

Sources. Most of the members of this complicated family of vitamins occur together in nature. For example they are present in the cells of both animal and vegetable tissues and are essential to the metabolic needs of the body. They are found especially in yeast, seeds (pea, bean and lentil), in eggs and in cereals such as wheat and rice. Some of the members of the group can also be prepared synthetically.

The most important are:

Vitamin B_1 or Aneurine, 'Thiamine.'

Vitamin B_2 or Riboflavine.

Vitamin B_3 or Nicotinic acid amide, Nicotinamide (niacin).

Vitamin B_6 or Pyridoxine.

Vitamin B_{12} or Cyanocobalamin (the extrinsic antianaemic factor).

Other substances in this group include pantothenic acid, folic acid and biotin (vitamin H).

Aneurine (Vitamin B_1)

Severe deficiency results in beri-beri, a disease affecting the nerves (peripheral neuritis). This mainly occurs among the rice-eating populations of the East where the staple diet is polished rice.

Minor degrees of deficiency may occur either due to lack of intake or to poor absorption. The latter may take place when the normal bacterial content of the intestines is altered by the prolonged administration of antibiotics by mouth and inadequate intake may occur in chronic alcoholism.

N.B.—Broad-spectrum antibiotics, e.g. tetracycline, may interfere with the absorption of vitamin B_1 from the gut.

In treatment the vitamin may be administered either by mouth or intramuscular injection (25 to 100 mg daily).

TABLE 5.—VITAMINS

Vitamins	Names	Sources	Effects	Notes
A	*Axerophthol*	Milk butter cream egg-yolk cod-liver oil spinach tomato carrots	Raises resistance to infection Prevents night-blindness Prevents eye disease (xerophthalmia)	Found in vegetables as carotene, converted into vitamin A in wall of small intestine
B	*Aneurine* or *Thiamine* Anti-neuritic	Peas beans lentils wholemeal bread husks of cereals (rice, wheat, oats, barley) yeast raw carrot cabbage	Prevents beri-beri Helps in treatment of alcoholic neuritis	*Riboflavine* is also associated with these vitamins and is called vitamin B_2 *Cyanocobalamin* is vitamin B_{12}, the intrinsic anti-anaemic factor
	Nicotinic acid amide		Prevents pellagra	
C	*Ascorbic acid* Anti-scorbutic	Acid fruits: orange lemon grape-fruit tomato cabbage swede	Prevents scurvy	Easily destroyed by heat and alkalis
D	*Calciferol* Anti-rachitic	Cod-liver oil eggs butter milk cream	Prevents rickets Necessary for calcium absorption	Also manufactured in the body by the action of sunlight (ultra-violet rays) on the skin
E	*Tocopheryl acetate*	Wheat germ oil	Prevents abortion	—
K	*Menaphthone*	Liver spinach other vegetables	Necessary for production of prothrombin	Antidote to 'Dindevan' over-dosage (K_1)
P	*Hesperidin Rutin*	Rose hips lemon juice	Affects permeability of capillaries	—

Riboflavine (Vitamin B$_2$)

Deficiency of this vitamin is associated with soreness of the lips and tongue and the development of fissures at the angle of the mouth. The average dose is 5 to 15 mg daily.

Nicotinc acid amide

Pellagra, a disease causing intestinal upset, skin eruptions, nervous symptoms and mental changes is due to lack of this vitamin. This also is a tropical disease not seen in this country in its fully developed form. Nicotinic acid is sometimes used as a vasodilator in a number of conditions but its effect is uncertain. It is also sometimes used to reduce serum cholesterol levels when they are abnormally high. Doses vary from 50 to 500 mg daily.

Cyanocobalamin (Vitamin B$_{12}$) is the extrinsic antianaemic factor used in the treatment of pernicious anaemia (p. 99).

Folic acid is used in the treatment of tropical sprue, coeliac disease and certain types of macrocytic anaemia. Dose 5 to 20 mg.

Vitamin C (Ascorbic acid—the anti-scorbutic vitamin)

Sources. This is found in fresh foodstuffs, especially fruits such as oranges, lemons, black currants, rose hips, tomatoes and green vegetables, and is therefore present in salads. It is rapidly destroyed by heat and is consequently lacking in tinned foods and boiled or dried milk.

Effects. Deficiency results in scurvy, a disease which may affect either infants or adults. It is characterized by haemorrhages into the tissues, under the skin and from the gums.

Ascorbic acid may also be a factor in the formation of haemo-globin and is sometimes given at the same time as iron in the treatment of anaemia. It can also act as a diuretic in the treatment of oedema in heart failure. It is given by mouth in doses of 50 to 100 mg three times daily.

Vitamin D (the anti-rachitic vitamin—Calciferol)

Sources. This is a very important vitamin and is more complicated than some of the others because it has two distinct sources:

(*a*) Its natural distribution especially in cod-liver oil (*oleum morrhuae*), and, to some extent, in butter and eggs.

(*b*) The body is able to manufacture it for itself by the action of sunlight on a steroid substance in the skin called 7-dehydro-cholesterol.

It is the ultra-violet rays of sunlight which have this action and, therefore, "artificial sunlight" has the same effect.

Effects. Lack of vitamin D causes rickets, a disease of young children characterized by deformities of the bones which are deficient in calcium. It plays an important part in the calcium metabolism of the body and its proper absorption from the intestine.

Prolonged high dosage is dangerous and may lead to the deposition of calcium in the kidneys and other organs.

The dosage varies from 1500 to 100,000 units daily.

Vitamin E (Tocopheryl acetate)

This is present in the germ of wheat and its deficiency is said to result in a tendency to abortion in early pregnancy and it may possibly have some effect on the nervous system. It has no established use in general medicine.

Vitamin K (Menaphthone)

This vitamin complex, which has been further subdivided into K_1 and K_2, is present in liver, spinach and other green vegetables. It is apparently necessary for the production of prothrombin (p. 108) in the body and, therefore, its deficiency results in a tendency to increased bleeding. It is given in some cases of jaundice, especially before operations and in neo-natal haemorrhage. Bile salts, which aid its absorption, are given at the same time in cases of obstructive jaundice. Synthetic preparations having the same action include menaphthone (1 to 10 milligrams by intramuscular injection) and acetomenaphthone (5 to 20 milligrams by mouth).

Vitamin K_1 acts especially as an antidote to overdosage with the anticoagulant drugs such as 'Dindevan' but not heparin. (1–10 mg are given by mouth, subcutaneously or intravenously.)

Vitamin P

Little is known about this vitamin group, but the functions of the capillaries appear to be influenced by it. Rutin and hesperidin have vitamin P activity.

Vitamin preparations

There are a number of "official" and even more proprietary vitamin preparations available. In many instances, more than one vitamin may be included in a preparation. The doses of the vitamins may be prescribed in units or by weight in milligrams.

A: Strong tablets of vitamin A ('Ro-A-Vit') 50,000 units.

B: Aneurine hydrochloride (*Aneurinae hydrochloridum*), 25–100 mg, available as tablets or an injection.
Nicotinic acid (*Acidum nicotinicum*) up to 500 milligrams.
Riboflavine (*Lactoflavin*) up to 15 milligrams.
'Bemax', 'Marmite', 'Benerva' and 'Becosym' are proprietary preparations containing vitamin B complex.

C: Ascorbic acid (*Acidum ascorbicum*), up to 500 milligrams.
Syrups of black currant and rose hips are rich sources of vitamin C, especially useful for children.

D: Calciferol and *Liquor calciferolis*.
Prophylactic: 10–20 micrograms, (400–800 units).
Therapeutic: 0·125–5·0 mg (500–200,000 units).

E: Tocopheryl acetate, up to 200 milligrams. 'Ephynal'.

K: Menaphthone, 'Synkavit', 'Konakion'.

Substances and preparations containing mixed vitamins include:
A and D: Cod-liver oil emulsion (*Emulsio olei morrhuae*), 8 to 30 ml. daily in divided doses.
In addition to the oil various emulsions are available which are designed to obscure its fishy taste.
Halibut liver oil capsules (*Caps. olei hippoglossi*), 1 to 3 capsules daily.
Vitamins A and D capsules (N.F.) (A = 4500, D = 450 units)
Vitamins A, B, C, and D are contained in Vitamins Capsules (N.F.), 'Multivite'.

Many proprietary vitamin preparations are available but only a few can be mentioned here.

Massive doses of mixed vitamin B complex with vitamin C (e.g. 'Orovite') are sometimes used in the treatment of toxic states, delirium tremens, acute alcoholism, barbiturate overdosage and acute mental conditions. Preparations for intravenous and intramuscular injection are available, e.g. 'Parentrovite'.

DRUGS USED IN METABOLIC DISORDERS

DIABETES

Diabetes is a disease due to deficiency of insulin normally secreted by the islets of Langerhans in the pancreas. It might therefore be regarded as an endocrine disorder, but its main feature is a disturbance of carbohydrate and, to some extent, fat metabolism. Normally, sugar (glucose) can only be utilized and fully oxidized by the tissues in the presence of insulin. If this is deficient, then sugar will accumulate in the blood and some of the excess will be excreted by the kidneys in the urine (glycosuria).

Further, it is only when sugar is being oxidized in the body, that an equivalent amount of fat can be fully broken down into carbon dioxide and water. If sugar is not being properly used by the tissues owing to lack of insulin, the breaking down of fat ceases at the fatty acid stage and diacetic acid and acetone (ketones) appear in the urine. The accumulation of ketones in the blood is called ketosis and ultimately leads to diabetic coma.

Diabetes may be controlled (a) by diet, (b) by insulin, (c) by oral hypoglycaemic agents or (d) some combination of these.

Insulin

The discovery of insulin has enabled the majority of diabetics to lead a normal life and to enjoy an interesting even though restricted diet. In many cases the patient can learn to give his own injections, test his own urine, and often adjust his diet to his daily requirements. The risk of diabetic coma has been very greatly reduced, but the possibilities of insulin over-dosage must not be forgotten.

Four types of insulin are commonly employed:

1. Soluble insulin.
2. Protamine zinc insulin.
3. Globin insulin.
4. Insulin zinc suspension. (Insulin lente).

Each of these may be used alone or a dose of soluble insulin may be needed in addition to protamine zinc or globin insulin, but not to insulin zinc suspension.

Soluble insulin is rapidly absorbed and has its maximum effect in about four to six hours.

Protamine zinc insulin acts more slowly. It has little action immediately after injection, but has its greatest effect in sixteen to eighteen hours.

Globin insulin comes between the other two with a maximum effect at twelve hours.

Insulin zinc suspension (lente) is a mixture of special types of short-acting (semilente or amorphous) and long-acting (ultralente or crystalline) insulins which is administered in a single morning dose and exerts its influence over the whole 24 hours in a manner

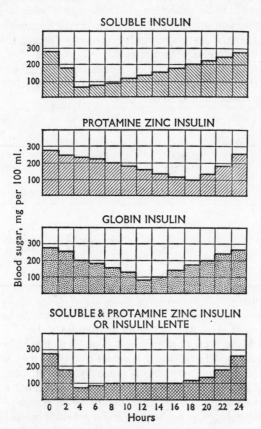

FIG. 6.—The effect of a dose of the various types of insulin on the blood sugar of a diabetic patient.

similar to the mixture of soluble and protamine zinc insulin. Insulin zinc suspension must not be mixed with other types of insulin and should probably not be used if the total dose required is high and if the patient shows a marked tendency to ketosis.

The aim in every case is to reduce the number of injections to one in twenty-four hours if possible, so that the dose and type of insulin must be carefully selected for each individual.

The various types of insulin are supplied in vials containing 20, 40 or 80 units per ml., and it is most important for both the nurse and the patient to be quite sure which strength is being used. In the case of protamine zinc and globin insulin the bottle must be shaken gently so that the suspended matter is evenly diffused throughout the mixture before any is withdrawn.

A patient ordered 20 units of insulin would be given 1 ml. of ordinary strength insulin, or ½ ml. of double strength, or ¼ ml. of quadruple strength, and so on.

TABLE 6.

Units	Single strength		Double strength		Quadruple strength	
	ml.	minims	ml.	minims	ml.	minims
10	0·5	8	0·25	4	—	—
20	1	16	0·5	8	0·25	4
30	1·5	25	0·75	12	0·38	6
40	2	33	1	16	0·5	8
50	2·5	40	1·25	20	0·62	10
100	5	80	2·5	40	1·25	20

The above table gives the approximate amounts to be injected when different strengths of insulin are employed.

Insulin keeps well if stored in a cool, dark place, but soluble insulin should not be used if it becomes cloudy. It may be administered with an ordinary hypodermic syringe or one specially graduated in units. This is kept in a metal case filled with spirit and may be rinsed in boiled water before use. It is wise to keep one needle for piercing the rubber cap and a separate one for injecting the insulin as the rubber is apt to cause blunting. The top of the rubber cap having been cleansed with spirit the requisite amount of insulin is drawn into the syringe. A small amount of air injected into the insulin bottle facilitates the removal of the liquid. The skin is cleaned with spirit or ether and the injection given subcutaneously. It may be made into the arms, thighs or abdomen—the latter sites being chosen if the patient is administering it himself.

Soluble insulin is given $\frac{1}{2}$ hour before a meal which must contain some carbohydrate food. The other types are given before breakfast.

While the process of standardization of insulin and diet is going on, the urine must be tested for sugar and acetone before each meal. When the regular dose of insulin has been determined daily tests should be carried out on the morning specimen.

The dose of insulin generally requires to be increased if the patient is suffering from any infection (e.g. a boil, severe cold, bronchitis, etc.).

It must be clearly understood that insulin is not a cure for the disease and, once being necessary, it is probable that the patient will have to continue taking it for the rest of his life, adjustments in the dosage being required from time to time.

Because of their delayed action protamine zinc insulin, zinc suspension (lente) and globin insulin should not be used in diabetic coma.

Unless the dose is carefully adjusted, protamine zinc and globin insulin are very liable to produce hypoglycaemia.

Other uses of insulin

(a) Small doses of insulin are sometimes given in order to increase the appetite in under-nourished patients.

(b) Large doses are used to produce a state of shock associated with hypoglycaemia in the treatment of certain mental cases (schizophrenia).

Oral hypoglycaemic agents

Patients on these agents should adhere to a strict diet calculated to maintain the normal weight for their height, sex and age.

(a) The sulphonylureas

These act by stimulating the islet cells of the pancreas to produce insulin and, therefore, can only be effective if the pancreas is capable of responding.

Tolbutamide ('Rastinon'). This substance is an oral anti-diabetic drug which lowers the blood sugar and may abolish glycosuria. It is most likely to be of use in the middle-aged diabetic in whom the disease is mild and of recent onset. In such cases the use of insulin injections may be avoided. It is unsuitable for juveniles, in diabetic coma and when there is liability to ketosis.

Dosage: 0·5–1·5 G daily in two or three divided doses.

Chlorpropamide ('Diabinese') has a similar action and use but is given in smaller doses, viz. 100 mg up to a maximum of 500 mg once daily with breakfast.

Side-effects such as nausea, vomiting and headache may occur and intolerance of alcohol may develop. Rarely jaundice or a skin rash is seen and indicates that the drug must be stopped at once.

Others include **tolazamide** ('Tolanase'), 100–500 mg; **aceto-hexamide** ('Dimelor'), 250–750 mg, **glymidine** ('Gondafon') 500 mg and **glibenclamide** ('Daonil') 5 mg.

Equivalent dosages 1·5G tolbutamide = 500 mg chlorpropamide = 5 mg glibenclamide.

(b) The diguanides

These compounds differ from the sulphonylureas in their mode of action, which is incompletely known. They may be used alone or in conjunction with insulin or a sulphonylurea. Used as sole therapy for diabetes, high doses cause gastrointestinal upsets. Occasionally, a serious acidosis (without hyperglycaemia) results from diguanide-therapy.

Phenformin ('Dibotin'). Dose: 50–300 mg daily.

Metformin ('Glucophage'). Dose: 1–3 G daily.

These drugs are taken in divided dosage, 2–3 times a day, after meals.

OBESITY

Obesity, an excess of body fat, is the commonest form of mal-nutrition in the Western world. It can cause some diseases (e.g. diabetes mellitus) and make others worse (e.g. heart disease and osteoarthritis).

The first approach to the treatment of obesity should be dietary. If the patient can be persuaded to eat less food than he requires for his daily energy expenditure, he will lose weight. The essence of a reducing diet is that it is low in calorific value. As most of a person's calories normally come from carbohydrates (sugar, flour products, potatoes, rice, etc) it is these which have to be reduced particularly. Few people eat too much protein or fat, partly because these are more expensive and partly because they are less palatable.

A number of drugs (anorectics) have been used to suppress appetite. The amphetamines were used for this purpose but many people became addicted to them because they had a stimulant effect on the central nervous system. They have therefore fallen into disfavour.

One drug which does not excite the central nervous system, and is not addictive, is **fenfluramine** ('Ponderax'). It causes an increase in the muscle uptake of glucose and has a fat-mobilizing action. The dose is 2 to 6 tablets daily, the dose being built up gradually. The drug is contraindicated in patients taking MAO inhibitors. Patients taking sedatives, antihypertensive drugs or hypoglycaemic agents may have to have the doses of these reduced when fenfluramine is administered.

GOUT

Gout is an obscure disorder of metabolism which results in the accumulation of uric acid in the blood and its deposition in the form of salts (urates) in and around joints, producing recurrent attacks of acute arthritis.

(a) Used during acute attack

Colchicum

This is the corm of a plant. The drug relieves acute attacks of gout. It has an irritating effect on the alimentary tract, causing vomiting and purgation.

It is usually given in the form of **colchicine** tablets, each containing 1 mg ($\frac{1}{60}$ grain) of the alkaloid colchicine. One mg is given, followed by 0·5 mg every two hours by mouth until the acute pain subsides or diarrhoea occurs.

An acute attack of gout will also respond to phenylbutazone, 200 mg two or three times daily. Corticosteroids are effective but are not recommended for routine use.

(b) Used between attacks

A number of compounds cause increased urinary excretion of uric acid. They are used (for the remainder of the patient's life) to reduce the number of acute attacks of gout, to reduce the size of tophi and to minimize renal damage. Drugs used are **salicylates**, e.g. sodium salicylate 6 G daily, **probenecid** ('Benemid') 0·5–2 G daily, **ethebenecid** ('Urelim') 0·5–1·5 G daily and **sulphinpyrazone** ('Anturan') 200–400 mg daily. Ample fluids, and often alkalis, should be taken to prevent urate deposition in the kidneys. These drugs are contraindicated in the presence of existing renal calculi.

Allopurinol ('Zyloric') restores serum uric acid levels to normal by diminishing the production of uric acid in the body. Less uric acid consequently passes through the kidneys and the drug therefore helps to prevent renal damage and uric acid stone formation. Dose: 200–600 mg daily in divided doses.

Salicylates antagonize the action of probenecid and sulphin-pyrazone and should not, therefore, be administered concurrently with them.

CHAPTER 15

The Ductless Glands and their Products

The ductless glands or endocrine organs are those glandular structures which pour their secretions (containing hormones) directly into the blood. A number of hormones have been isolated and some can be prepared in the laboratory. The functions of all the ductless glands are intimately connected with each other and also with the nervous system. The pituitary gland, in particular, exercises control over the suprarenals, thyroid, pancreas and sex glands. They play an important part in the metabolic processes of the body and in growth. Because of the balance which exists between the activities of the various glands, a disorder of one may upset the functions of others.

In a broad sense, disordered function of a ductless gland may result either in an increase or a decrease in the amount of its secretion. The various ductless gland products employed in therapeutics may be used either to substitute for a deficiency due to undersecretion of the gland, or in order to influence the activity of other glands or organs.

The substances used may be:

(i) The actual gland substance itself.

(ii) Specially prepared extracts from the gland.

(iii) Chemically prepared substances identical with or closely resembling the natural hormone.

(iv) In certain instances, some hormones can be extracted from the urine.

THE THYROID GLAND

The internal secretion of the thyroid is found in the colloid material secreted by the epithelium lining the vesicles of the gland. Its active principles are thyroxine and triiodothyronine (liothyronine), hormones with high iodine contents.

Over-secretion of the thyroid gland produces thyrotoxicosis (exophthalmic goitre or Graves' disease). Among the effects of this disease is a general increase in metabolism so that the individual tends to lose weight. Under-secretion results in myxoedema in the adult, and cretinism in the infant.

Preparations of thyroid are used for the following purposes:

1. In myxoedema and cretinism, because the secretion is defective. In such cases, the patient must continue to take appropriate doses for the rest of his life.

2. In some cases of non-toxic (simple) goitre.

Excessive dosage produces symptoms resembling thyrotoxicosis, the most important being marked loss of weight, sweating and a rapid pulse.

Preparations

Thyroid (*Thyroideum*), 30–250 mg ($\frac{1}{2}$ to 4 grains) daily.

This is obtained by extracting the dried gland of animals such as oxen, sheep and pigs. It is usually supplied in tablets containing $\frac{1}{2}$ grain. (1 gr. thyroid approximates 0·1 thyroxine).

Various proprietary extracts are also available, e.g. 'Elityran'. It is given by mouth and, in fact, thyroid is the only gland substance which can be given effectively in this way.

Thyroxine sodium ('Eltroxin')

This very powerful synthetic substance, resembling the natural hormone, is now usually preferred to thyroid tablets. Dose: 0·05–0·5 mg daily. A dose of 0·1 mg is about equivalent to 60 mg of thyroid.

Liothyronine sodium ('Tertroxin') is more potent than thyroxine and its greater rapidity of action renders it useful for certain cases, e.g. myxoedematous madness.

Dose: 10–80 micrograms daily. Twenty micrograms is equivalent to 60 mg of thyroid.

Antithyroid substances

In cases of thyrotoxicosis it is necessary to diminish the activity of the thyroid gland. This may be done either by surgical removal of a considerable proportion of the gland or by the administration of a drug which suppresses its activity. In any event it is usual to give some medical treatment to patients before an operation is performed.

Iodine. This will temporarily depress the function of the thyroid but its maximum effect is reached after two weeks of administration after which it may be given for a further period of three weeks when it ceases to be effective. It is, therefore, only suitable as a pre- and immediate postoperative measure. Lugol's iodine (*Liquor iodi aquosus*), 0·3–1 ml. (5 to 15 minims), a watery solution of iodine with potassium, is generally employed, commencing with 2 minims and increasing to 5 or 10 minims three times a day. Potassium iodide in doses of 60 to 100 mg thrice daily may be used instead.

Radioactive iodine (^{131}I) may be used in the diagnosis of thyroid disease and sometimes in the treatment of thyrotoxicosis in patients over the age of 45 and in carcinoma of the thyroid. Cases are carefully selected and an appropriate dose is required for each of the uses mentioned. (p. 262)·

Carbimazole ('Neomercazole'), 30–45 mg daily in divided doses (maintenance 5–15 mg),

This is a drug which depresses the activity of the gland and can effect a medical cure of thyrotoxicosis in suitable cases. Symptoms may be controlled in one to three months but it is usually necessary to continue with a maintenance dose for one to two years. It may be two or three weeks before a therapeutic response is apparent.

It is less toxic than thiouracil but may also cause serious agranulocytosis and skin rashes.

Thiouracil. This is a sulphur-containing drug which has been used in the treatment of thyrotoxicosis in the form of methyl- or propyl-thiouracil. Although it does not have much effect on the protrusion of the eyes (exophthalmos) or the goitre, like carbimazole it restores the raised metabolism rate to normal and many patients are able to return to work after one to three months of treatment.

Toxic symptoms are sometimes produced. The most serious is diminution of the white blood cells (agranulocytosis): others include pyrexia, gland enlargement and rashes. Iodine should not be used at the same time.

Potassium perchlorate has been used as an anti-thyroid drug in doses of 200 mg four times daily when others are contraindicated. As a rule this dose may be halved after three or four weeks. Iodine containing drugs should not be given at the same time. Aplastic anaemia is a rare, but usually fatal, complication of therapy with this drug which is best avoided.

THE PARATHYROID GLANDS

Although anatomically so closely related to the thyroid gland, the function of the parathyroids is entirely different. They secrete a hormone, parathormone, the function of which is to control calcium metabolism in the body. An excess of it causes an increase in the serum calcium level. Another hormone, calcitonin, reduces the serum calcium level.

Deficiency of parathyroid secretion results in tetany, which is characterized by muscular spasms and increased irritability of the nervous system. The blood calcium is low. Tetany may occur, (*a*) after removal of the parathyroids, (*b*) in some cases of rickets, (*c*) after very large doses of alkali, (*d*) in sprue.

Increased activity of the parathyroids gives rise to a rare disease (hyperparathyroidism) in which there is loss of calcium from the bones. The calcium is lost into the urine where it may cause stone formation.

Preparation

Parathyroid ('Parathormone')

This must be given by injection. It is used for diagnostic purposes but is not now generally used for the treatment of parathyroid deficiency. The main reasons for this are:

(*a*) It acts too slowly to be of use in acute tetany.

(*b*) The body becomes refractory to its action if it is used for long-term treatment.

Calcium gluconate (10 ml. of 10% solution) given intravenously is the immediate treatment for tetany. In the long-term management of parathyroid deficiency, a diet low in phosphorus is recommended. This is supplemented by calcium salts, e.g. calcium lactate or gluconate (up to 20 G daily). Such treatment is adequate for mild cases but in more severe cases it is also necessary to give calciferol (vitamin D_2), usually in a dose of 100,000 units daily, by mouth. Alternatively, a chemically related substance, dihydro-tachysterol ('AT 10') may be given in a dose of 1 to 10 ml. daily, by mouth. This substance resembles parathyroid hormone in causing increased urinary excretion of phosphate.

THE SUPRARENAL OR ADRENAL GLANDS

The two suprarenal glands consist of an outer cortex and central medulla each of which produce hormones differing in chemical character and function. The glands are plentifully supplied with blood and also with sympathetic nerve fibres from the coeliac (solar) plexus.

The suprarenal cortex is essential to life and secretes a number of hormones, each having different functions. Some of these have been extracted from the gland and some can be made in the laboratory.

Chemically they belong to a class of fatty or wax-like substances called steroids or corticoids. The most important ones fall into three main groups:

1. The **Mineral Corticoids** of which deoxycortone (DOCA) and aldosterone are examples. These act on the tubules of the kidney in such a way that:

(a) sodium and chloride are retained in the body,

(b) excess of potassium is excreted.

They therefore help to maintain the water and electrolyte balance of the body. Any excess or overdosage will tend to cause water retention (oedema) and hypertension.

2. The **Gluco-corticoids** or **Corticosteroids**. This group includes cortisone and its derivatives. (For brevity the term "steroid" may be employed.) These hormones have a number of actions, one of the main ones being to influence carbohydrate and glucose metabolism.

(a) They assist in the conversion of carbohydrate into glycogen.

(b) They increase the blood sugar.

(c) They help in the utilization of fat.

(d) They decrease the number of lymphocytes and eosinophils in the blood.

(e) They reduce the rate at which certain connective tissue cells multiply and so tend to suppress the natural reaction to infection and to delay healing.

(f) They increase the secretion of hydrochloride acid in the stomach, thus tending to cause peptic ulcers or to delay their healing.

(g) In large doses cortisone produces symptoms similar to Cushing's syndrome, viz. a swollen, round "moon face", excess of hair and a tendency to acne.

(h) Electrolyte and water metabolism disturbances.

3. **Sex (Gonad-like) Hormones** similar to those produced by the

ovary and testis (oestrogens and androgens). These influence growth
and sex development.

The output of hormones from the cortex of the suprarenal is
controlled by another hormone secreted by the pituitary gland
known as the adreno-cortico-trophic hormone (ACTH) or corticotrophin. Unlike the medulla of the suprarenal the secretions of the
cortex are not regulated by nervous impulses.

Cortisone, hydrocortisone and many similar synthetic substances
(e.g. prednisone and prednisolone) are all used in clinical medicine.
When cortisone is administered in large doses among the complications observed is a disturbance of salt and water balance, due to
the fact that it has some mineralocorticoid effect in addition to its
glucocorticoid action.

It must also be remembered that although the individual hormones mentioned each have separate effects on metabolism, in
health, normal suprarenal cortical secretion represents the sum of
all these individual actions.

In disease, if the suprarenal cortex is destroyed or if the secretion
of corticotrophin (ACTH) fails there will be no suprarenal cortical
hormones produced.

Mineral corticoids

1. **Deoxycortone** (DOCA), 2–5 mg. This mineral corticoid which
causes water and sodium retention may be used in conjunction
with cortisone in the treatment of Addison's disease. Overdosage
produces oedema and hypertension.

(*a*) It may be given by intramuscular injection in doses of 2–5
mg daily.

(*b*) Pellets (100–400 mg) may be implanted under the skin
whence it is slowly absorbed over a period of about six months.

2. **Fludrocortisone** ('Florinef'). This synthetic salt-retaining
steroid has now largely replaced deoxycortone in the treatment of
Addison's disease. Its great advantage is that it is an oral medica-
tion.

Dose: 0·1–0·3 mg daily.

Deoxycortone remains of value in patients who are vomiting or
cannot, for some reason, take tablets.

3. **Aldosterone**, the main natural salt-retaining steroid, is not
commercially available.

Gluco-corticoids (Corticosteroids)

Cortisone 50–400 mg

Since cortisone was originally discovered a number of other substances having a similar general action have been made by varying slightly its chemical composition. By means of these variations it has been possible to minimize some of the side-effects so that prednisone and prednisolone cause less salt and water retention particularly as they can be given in one fifth of the dose of cortisone. The more recent synthetic steroids, methyl prednisolone, triamcinolone, dexamethasone and betamethasone, have minimal salt-retaining effect. The latter two have thirty-five times the anti-inflammatory effect of cortisone. Prednisone and prednisolone are, however, generally the steroids of choice for systemic administration.

Hydrocortisone is the form in which the hormone is actually secreted in the body by the adrenal glands and its action is identical with that of cortisone.

There are a large number of proprietary preparations of these substances each having different names and too numerous to mention here.

The cortisone group of drugs may be used as tablets, injections, ointments and eye drops.

(*a*) Cortisone, prednisone and prednisolone are used mainly for internal administration.

(*b*) Hydrocortisone, although it can be given internally and, in grave emergency, by intravenous injection, is used mainly for local application and local injection into and around joints.

Cortisone (50–400 mg), **prednisone and prednisolone** 5–100 mg daily) etc.

These substances may be used either as direct replacement therapy, i.e. to replace the natural hormone when the secretion of the adrenal gland is defective as in Addison's disease or after removal of both glands (which may be performed for certain cases of carcinoma, e.g. of the breast) or empirically, where increase of the cortical steroid hormones has been shown by experiment to be beneficial.

Among the many conditions in which they may be used are:

1. *Rheumatic and collagen diseases*
   rheumatic fever   polyarteritis nodosa   acute gout
   rheumatoid arthritis   lupus erythematosus

2. *Allergic disorders*
  severe asthma   drug sensitivity   status asthmaticus
                                                serum sickness

3. *Skin diseases*
  pemphigus vulgaris   dermatitis   erythema
                                                  multiforme

4. *Endocrine disorders*
  Addison's disease   pituitary disorders   adrenalectomy

5. *Blood diseases*
  haemolytic anaemia   purpura

6. *Other disorders*
  ulcerative colitis   temporal arteritis   nephrotic
  burns   sarcoidosis   syndrome
                                                delirium tremens

There are a number of other uncommon conditions in which the use of cortisone may be considered desirable. It must be understood, however, that it is only used in selected cases and is not necessarily employed in every case of the diseases listed.

Contraindications. Being a very powerful drug cortisone must be used with great caution and under careful supervision. It is usually contraindicated in the presence of peptic ulcer, hypertension and cardiac insufficiency, and in most cases of active or old tuberculosis although there are special indications for its use in some cases of tuberculosis.

In view of the fact that the administration of cortisone tends to inhibit the natural secretion from the adrenal gland while it is being given the drug should be withdrawn gradually over a period of several weeks when therapy has been completed otherwise serious withdrawal symptoms may occur.

When cortisone is given in large doses the following observations are desirable:

(*a*) Daily weight, urinary output and blood pressure records.

(*b*) Observation for oedema, "moon face" and thrombophlebitis of legs.

(*c*) Diet: high protein, restricted fat and carbohydrate.

(*d*) Drugs:

  potassium chloride to prevent potassium depletion;
  aluminium hydroxide to prevent peptic ulcer;

antibiotics in the presence of infection;
sedatives to minimize mental disturbances.

These precautions are less necessary when prednisone and prednisolone are used unless large doses are employed.

Hydrocortisone. This may be injected with strict aseptic precautions into or around joints. Doses of 0·25–1 ml. (25 mg per ml.)
are used according to the size of the joint or area to be infiltrated.

Among the conditions for which it may be employed are:

rheumatoid arthritis	traumatic arthritis
osteoarthritis	"tennis elbow"
periarthritis	acute gout
bursitis	keloid scars

Retention enemas may be given in ulcerative colitis, e.g. 50–100
mg in 150 ml. of 1% methyl cellulose emulsion or normal saline
once or twice daily.

Hydrocortisone lotion and skin ointment

Lotions are generally used for wet surfaces and extensive lesions,
ointments for dry localized lesions and those near the eyes. At first
applications may be made up to four times daily and later reduced
to daily or alternate days. Among the indications are:

allergic skin disorders	pruritus
eczema of various types	contact dermatitis

Hydrocortisone eye drops (1%) and eye ointment (2·5%)

blepharitis	interstitial keratitis
conjunctivitis	iritis

Their use is contraindicated in acute corneal ulcer.

FUNCTIONS OF ADRENAL MEDULLA

The medulla secretes adrenaline, the properties of which have
already been mentioned (p. 164); they include:

(i) It is a general stimulant of the sympathetic system.

(ii) It is a vasoconstrictor.

(iii) It raises blood pressure.

(iv) It causes the liver to liberate glucose from glycogen.

The medulla also secretes noradrenaline, (p. 165) a natural
hormone closely related to adrenaline which can also be prepared
synthetically. It also raises blood pressure by vasoconstriction but
has little effect on the bronchial muscle.

A rare tumour of the adrenal medulla (phoeochromocytoma) is a cause of hypertension, because of the noradrenaline and adrenaline which it secretes.

THE PITUITARY GLAND

This consists of two parts which have different modes of development and entirely different functions.

1. *Anterior lobe.* This secretes a number of hormones having the following functions:

(*a*) The growth hormone (somatotrophin).

(*b*) The thyrotropic or thyroid stimulating hormone (TTH or TSH). This appears to stimulate the growth and activity of the thyroid gland and to increase the basal metabolic rate.

(*c*) The adreno-cortico-trophic hormone (ACTH). This hormone is a protein substance which stimulates the cortex of the suprarenal gland to secrete its own hormones, e.g.:

(i) Mineral steroids (corticoids) e.g. deoxycortone (DOCA) and aldosterone, to a minor extent.

(ii) Gluco-steroids e.g. cortisone, etc. (p. 201).

(*d*) The gonado-trophic hormones. These are essential for the normal development of the sex organs and stimulate the production of the various sex gland hormones. They are:

(i) The follicle stimulating hormone (FSH). In the female this stimulates the ripening of the ovarian follicles. In the male it stimulates the production of spermatozoa.

(ii) The luteinizing hormone (LH). In the female this stimulates rupture of the follicles (ovulation) and formation of corpora lutea. Acting with FSH, it stimulates oestrogen production. Acting with prolactin, it stimulates progesterone production in the corpus luteum. In the male, it stimulates the testes to produce testosterone.

(*e*) The lactogenic hormone (prolactin, luteotrophin) which helps to control the secretion of milk from the breast. It also maintains the secretory activity of the corpus luteum.

Adreno-cortico-trophic hormone (ACTH), corticotrophin

ACTH is a hormone obtained from the anterior lobe of the pituitary gland used in therapeutics. Its action is to stimulate the cortex of the suprarenal gland to produce various hormones, the most important of which is cortisone. (p. 200).

The effect of cortisone can, therefore, be produced either by its own direct administration or by giving ACTH which stimulates its production in the body.

They may be used in diseases affecting the respective glands, i.e. ACTH may be given in hypopituitarism and cortisone in Addison's disease. In practice, however, cortisone is prescribed for both conditions. Cortisone and ACTH also have effects in many other conditions.

ACTH is given by intramuscular injection in doses of 10 to 25 units at six hourly intervals. Gelatin preparations which delay absorption are also available so that only a daily injection is necessary.

Tetracosactrin is a synthetic substance which stimulates the adrenal cortex as ACTH does. It is available in a short-acting form ('Synacthen'), used mainly for diagnostic purposes, and in a long-acting form ('Synacthen Depot') which acts for up to 48 hours and is therefore used therapeutically. The dose of the long-acting preparation is 0·5 to 1 mg intramuscularly, perhaps daily at first and later twice a week.

Anterior lobe preparations

ACTH has long been prepared, for therapeutic use, from the anterior lobe of animal pituitary glands. Human growth hormone (HGH) is available, in short supply, for the treatment of hypopituitary dwarfs. FSH has also been extracted from human pituitary glands and used in the treatment of infertility. Growth hormone and FSH of animal origin are ineffective in the human subject.

Substances having an action on the gonads or sex glands similar to that produced by the anterior pituitary hormones can be obtained from the placenta and urine of pregnant women and mares. These are called **gonadotrophic hormones** and are sometimes used in the treatment of menorrhagia, dysmenorrhoea and sterility in the female. In the male they may be used for undescended testicle and some cases of impotence. In all cases their effects are variable and uncertain.

1. Chorionic gonadotrophin (from urine of pregnant women). Dose: 500–1000 units, twice weekly, intramuscularly. Proprietary preparations include 'Pregnyl', 'Gonan'. The action resembles LH.

2. Serum gonadotrophin (from serum of pregnant mares). Dose: 200–1000 units, twice weekly, intramuscularly. The action resembles a mixture of LH and FSH.

The patient's own pituitary gland may often be stimulated to secrete gonadotrophins by administering a synthetic drug known as **clomiphene** ('Clomid'). This effect may be used to induce ovulation and thereby to make pregnancy possible in some women who are infertile because of ovarian dysfunction (failure to ovulate). Multiple births sometimes result from clomiphene therapy and the treatment should be supervised by a doctor with special experience.

Posterior lobe preparations

Extracts of the posterior lobe which contain two active substances:

1. **Oxytocin** ('Pitocin'). This is used in obstetrics, to cause contraction of the uterus without increasing the blood pressure.

(i) To induce labour.

(ii) In the second stage of labour, when the os is fully dilated, to overcome uterine inertia.

(iii) In the prophylaxis and treatment of post-partum haemorrhage.

(iv) To aid the expulsion of the placenta or retained products from the uterus after delivery.

(v) To stimulate uterine contraction during the operation of Caesarean section, immediately after the infant and the placenta have been removed. In this instance it is sometimes injected directly into the uterine muscle.

Dose: Injection of oxytocin (B.P.) 2–5 units. This is given by slow intravenous infusion (in 1 litre of 5 per cent dextrose solution), intramuscularly or subcutaneously. It is also prepared in a tablet (200 units) for absorption in the mouth.

2. **Vasopressin** ('Pitressin') which has the following actions:

(*a*) To raise blood pressure by acting on the plain muscles of the arteries producing vaso-constriction.

(*b*) To cause contraction of plain muscle, especially of the intestines and bladder.

(*c*) An anti-diuretic action causing water retention in the body. Use is made of this property in the treatment of diabetes insipidus, in which it may be administered by injection or in the form of snuff.

Dose: Injection of vasopressin (B.P.) 2–5 units.

'**Pituitrin**' is a proprietary preparation containing both substances and therefore has the following actions:

(*a*) Those due to oxytocin ('Pitocin')—see above.

(*b*) Those due to vasopressin ('Pitressin') which stimulates plain muscle:

(i) It increases peristalsis in the intestines and is used in cases of paralytic ileus and postoperative distension.

(ii) To cause vasoconstriction by acting on the plain muscle in the arteries and so to raise blood pressure. It is not recommended for this purpose, however, because it may cause dangerous constriction of the coronary arteries.

(iii) On account of other actions it is sometimes used in diabetes insipidus, haemoptysis, herpes zoster.

THE SEX GLANDS

The hormones used in therapy may be divided into two main groups:

1. Female sex hormones derived from the ovary.

2. Male sex hormones derived from the testis.

Some synthetic preparations are also available.

1. The internal secretions of the ovary

Two main types of preparation are used:

(*a*) Oestrogens.

(*b*) Progesterone and synthetic progestational compounds (progestogens).

(a) Oestrogens

These are substances which produce the effects of the hormone of the ovarian follicle including:

(i) Development of the female secondary sexual characteristics, i.e. growth of pubic and axillary hair, the breasts and external genitalia.

(ii) Rhythmic contraction of the Fallopian tube and its fimbriae which collect the ovum at the time of ovulation.

(iii) Growth of the uterine muscle and endometrium.

(iv) Secretion from the glands of the cervix.

(v) The smoothness of the female skin in comparison with the greasy skin of the male.

The main uses are:

(i) To diminish unpleasant symptoms occurring at the menopause.

(ii) To suppress lactation on weaning or after a stillbirth, e.g. stilboestrol, 15 mg, t.d.s. for three days combined with a diuretic.

(iii) In certain cases of excessive uterine bleeding (metropathia haemorrhagica).

(iv) In some cases of amenorrhoea.

(v) In senile vaginitis and kraurosis vulvae.

(vi) In some cases of carcinoma of the prostate in males and of the breast in females.

(vii) In some cases of acne both in the male and female.

Toxic effects include:

(i) Nausea and vomiting.

(ii) Excessive uterine bleeding especially after the drug is withdrawn.

There are two main types of oestrogen:

(i) Natural: obtained from human sources or from the urine of pregnant mares: e.g. oestrone, oestradiol, 'Premarin'.

(ii) Synthetic: e.g. stilboestrol, dienoestrol, ethinyloestradiol, methallenoestril.

Generally speaking the former are expensive and the latter relatively cheap (especially stilboestrol).

The doses vary according to the preparation and the purpose for which it is given. Oral administration is usually effective but preparations for intramuscular injection are available. Many proprietary preparations are on the market. 'Menopax' cream, used locally for pruritus vulvae, contains stilboestrol, amethocaine and benzocaine.

(b) Progesterone

This is a hormone formed mainly by the cells of the corpus luteum which develop in the ovarian follicle after the ovum has been extruded. Its main action is to sensitize the endometrium and prepare it for the reception of the fertilized ovum. It also relaxes plain muscle, which may contribute to the occurrence of varicose veins, constipation and dilation of the ureters during pregnancy.

Its main use is when combined with oestrogen in the treatment of menstrual disorders and in the treatment of excessive uterine bleeding. Its effects in the treatment of abortion and sterility are uncertain. Preparations are given by intramuscular injection in the form of an oily solution.

Ethisterone and other synthetic preparations are given by mouth. Progestogen/oestrogen mixtures (e.g. 'Anovlar 21',

'Conovid', 'Norlestrin', 'Ortho-Novin') are used for fertility control. Side-effects include amenorrhoea, nausea, headaches and thromboembolic complications.

2. The male sex hormones (Androgens)

Testosterone

This is an active substance which is obtained from the testes and which can also be prepared chemically.

Various compounds of testosterone may be given by intramuscular injection or by implantation under the skin. Methyltestosterone is given by mouth.

Main uses:

1. Male hypogonadism and after castration.

2. In a number of gynaecological conditions including excessive uterine bleeding, endometriosis and premenstrual tension.

Testosterone may produce excessive growth of facial hair in the female and salt and water retention leading to oedema.

3. In disseminated carcinoma of the breast in post-menopausal women.

Anabolic steroids

One important property of testosterone is its stimulation of protein synthesis, i.e. its anabolic effect. Compounds have been developed which have the anabolic but only a fraction of the and rogenic effect of testosterone. They may therefore be used in women with less risk of inducing virilization. These drugs include norethandrolone ('Nilevar') and nandrolone ('Durabolin'). They are used to accelerate growth in some types of dwarf. They are also used in debilitating illnesses and osteoporosis. Their long-term value in the latter condition is very doubtful and so is calcium therapy.

ORAL CONTRACEPTION

This subject is closely connected with the use of hormone preparations. It does not involve the use of mechanical methods of contraception, intra-uterine devices, chemical spermicides or fertility control by periodic abstinence.

If oral contraceptives are taken according to direction they are practically 100 per cent effective in preventing pregnancy and have the advantage that aesthetic considerations are not involved. There may be, however, a few minor and even major side-effects.

There are two main types in use:

1. Preparations containing oestrogen and progestogen, taken for 22 consecutive days in each 28-day cycle.

2. Two sets of tablets, (*a*) those taken for the first 16 days of the cycle; (*b*) those taken for the last 5 to 7 days, containing both progestogen and oestrogen.

There are also preparations containing only progestogen which have not proved so reliable.

Minor side-effects. These include headache, temporary nausea, breast tenderness and occasional hypertension and depression.

Major side-effects. Fortunately these are rare but there is evidence that there is a slight increase in the incidence of venous thrombosis which may lead to fatal embolism. This must, however, be measured against the possible complications of pregnancy.

FERTILITY DRUGS

The use of these drugs is still largely experimental and in the hands of experts. Lack of fertility involves investigation both of the male and female partners in the first instance. At this stage of knowledge little if anything can be done to improve male infertility and lack of spermatogenesis. On the other hand, provided that the ovaries contain the necessary follicles there are preparations (e.g. clomiphene) which influence ovulation in the female. They may, however, lead to multiple births.

CHAPTER 16

Miscellaneous Drugs

DRUGS ACTING ON THE UTERUS

The uterus is an organ composed of plain muscle fibres and lined by a special type of mucous membrane, the endometrium. Its functions are (i) to receive the fertilized ovum and to retain the developing foetus throughout pregnancy, (ii) to expel the foetus and placenta at the end of pregnancy.

After puberty the endometrium undergoes a series of periodic changes by which it is prepared to receive a fertilized ovum at regular intervals of about a month. Menstruation is the process by which the specially prepared endomentrium is shed when no fertilized ovum has been received.

When the end of pregnancy is reached, the greatly hypertrophied muscle of the body of the uterus commences to contract in a succession of recurring spasms which gradually increase in frequency. At the same time the muscle of the cervix dilates, and when fully dilated the head of the foetus can descend to the perineum, whence the child is finally delivered. Some minutes later this is followed by the placenta and the membranes which surround the foetus during its development in the uterus.

Apart from the female sex hormones which may influence ovarian and uterine function, comparatively few drugs have any important action on the non-pregnant uterus.

On the other hand it must be remembered that some modern drugs may have a genetic effect on the foetus and careful consideration must be given before they are administered, e.g. cyto-toxic drugs. Drugs which cause foetal malformations are said to be **teratogenic.** All new drugs are tested for teratogenicity in animals. Unfortunately, absence of teratogenicity in animals does not guarantee safety for the human foetus. All new drugs are therefore used with great caution in women who may be in the early stages of pregnancy. In prescribing *any* drug for a pregnant woman the doctor has to be sure that it is essential.

Drugs which increase uterine contraction

The drugs which increase uterine contraction once labour is due or has commenced are called **ecbolics**.

There are no drugs which act on the uterus in the early stages of pregnancy which would cause it to expel its contents without producing poisonous symptoms dangerous to the life of the mother. In other words, there are no true abortifacients available which have any therapeutic use. If, for medical reasons, it is necessary to terminate pregnancy in the early stages, operative procedures must be carried out.

Ergot (*Ergota*)

This is a fungus which grows on rye and sometimes on other kinds of grain. Its action is due to the various alkaloids which it contains. It causes contraction of the muscle of the pregnant uterus during and after labour, and is, therefore, especially valuable:

(i) In the treatment of post-partum haemorrhage, when the contraction of the uterine muscle closes the bleeding vessels.

(ii) In aiding the expulsion of the placenta and any retained products of conception.

(ii) To keep the uterine muscle firmly contracted during the first few days of the puerperium.

The following preparations may be employed:

Ergometrine maleate

Ergot capsules and tablets, 150–500 mg ($2\frac{1}{2}$–$7\frac{1}{2}$ grains).

Ergometrine maleate. This is an alkaloid which is given in the following doses:

By mouth (tablets): 0·5–1 mg ($\frac{1}{120}$–$\frac{1}{60}$ grain).

By intramuscular injection: 0·25–1 mg ($\frac{1}{240}$–$\frac{1}{60}$ grain).

By intravenous injection: 0·125–0·5 mg ($\frac{1}{480}$–$\frac{1}{120}$ grain).

'Syntometrin' contains ergometrine and oxytocin.

Pituitary (posterior lobe)

It has already been noted (p. 206) that the extract of the posterior lobe of the pituitary contains **oxytocin** ('Pitocin') which causes the plain muscle of the pregnant uterus to contract without producing a rise in blood pressure. Subcutaneous or intramuscular dose, 2 to 5 units.

Pituitary (posterior lobe) (Injection, BPC, 0·2–0·5 ml., subcutaneously or intramuscularly, is now less often used than the pure hormone oxytocin (which may be prepared synthetically).

Quinine (*Quinina*)

Quinine is a drug having a number of actions (p. 220). Among them is the ability to cause labour to commence during the last weeks of pregnancy. It has been used in the "medical induction" of labour, but 'Pitocin' is now preferred for this purpose.

Uterine sedatives

These are substances which diminish the force and frequency of the muscular contractions of the pregnant uterus, e.g. morphine, chloral hydrate.

Halothane effectively relaxes the uterus during the time that it is being administered.

Diagnosis of uterine conditions

'Hypaque' may be injected into the uterine cavity. Normally, it fills this cavity and also the Fallopian tubes. An X-ray after the injection shows the outline of the uterus, its size and shape and also the patency of the tubes. This procedure may be of importance in the diagnosis of sterility and is called hystero-salpingography.

PREPARATIONS ACTING ON THE VAGINA

1. *Trichomonas* infection: Acetarsol pessaries. Metronidazole ('Flagyl') tablets, taken orally, 1 t.d.s. for 7 days.

2. *Monilia* infections: Crystal violet pessaries. Nystatin.

3. Antiseptic application: (*a*) Chloroxylenol irrigation, one tablespoonful of solution mixed with one pint of warm water, (*b*) Proflavine pessaries, (*c*) 'Penotrane' pessaries.

4. Astringent lotions: Zinc sulphate irrigation. Six grams in 500 ml. (90 grains in 1 pint) of warm water.

5. To alter acidity of vagina: Lactic acid pessary, Lactic acid irrigation. One tablespoonful in one pint of warm water.

6. For senile vaginitis: Stilboestrol pessary.

DRUGS ACTING ON THE EYE

Therapeutic substances may be applied to the eyes in the following types of preparation:

Eye lotions (*Collyria*).
Eye drops (*Guttae pro oculis*).⎫ For details see National
Eye ointments (*Oculenta*). ⎬ Formulary.
Gelatin discs (*Lamellae*). ⎭

1. Drugs which dilate the pupil (Mydriatics)

The most important are atropine and homatropine.

Atropine

Atropine dilates the pupil and paralyses the power of accommodation when given internally and when applied locally to the eye (p. 169). Locally, it takes several hours to produce its full effect, which lasts for several days. It has the disadvantage of increasing the tension within the eye and is, therefore, contraindicated in cases of glaucoma. It is used for the following purposes:

(i) In the treatment of iritis. By paralysing its power of movement the iris is rested.

(ii) in cases of corneal ulcer.

(iii) In injury to the eyeball.

(iv) For purposes of examination of the retina.

It may be applied in the form of drops, gelatin discs or an ointment.

Atropine sulphate drops (*Guttae atropinae sulphatis*), 1 per cent
Atropine discs (*Lamellae*), 0·013 mg.
Atropine eye ointment (*Oculentum atropinae*), 1 per cent.

These preparations are sometimes combined with cocaine for use in painful conditions.

Homatropine

This has a similar but much more rapid, though less prolonged, action than atropine. The pupils are dilated in 5 to 15 minutes and the effect passes off in a few hours.

Homatropine is especially useful for rapid dilation of the pupils prior to examination of the optic discs.

Drops (2 per cent) or gelatine discs may be employed. Ointments are also available, and cocaine may be added for the treatment of painful conditions.

It must be remembered that patients may not be able to see properly until the effects of atropine and homatropine have worn off. Reading will be impossible and they may find it very difficult to get about out of doors in bright light.

NORMAL

MORPHINE
(pin point)

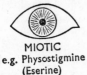

MIOTIC
e.g. Physostigmine
(Eserine)

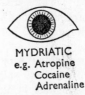

MYDRIATIC
e.g. Atropine
Cocaine
Adrenaline

Fig. 7.—Diagram illustrating the action of drugs on the pupil.

II. Drugs which contract the pupil (Miotics)

Physostigmine ('Eserine')

This is the most important miotic drug. It is used especially in the treatment of glaucoma and may be employed to counteract the effect of atropine and homatropine when eye examinations have been completed. In glaucoma, contraction of the iris helps to open up the lymph channels in the ciliary body, thereby facilitating the drainage of fluid from the interior of the eye and lowering intraocular tension. (See also p. 168).

Drops, gelatine discs and ointment may be used.

Physostigmine (Eserine') drops (*Guttae physostigminae*), 0·5 per cent.

Physostigmine ('Eserine') discs (*Lamellae physostigminae*) 0·065 mg ($\frac{1}{1000}$ grain).

Physostigmine ('Eserine') eye ointment (*Oculentum physostigminae*) (0·125 per cent).

Guanethedine ('Ismelin') eye drops are used in the treatment of chronic glaucoma and also in the exophthalmos of thyrotoxicosis.

Local anaesthetics

Cocaine drops, 2 per cent, are generally employed (*a*) for operations on the eye, (*b*) to render the conjunctiva anaesthetized in order that a foreign body may be removed and (*c*) in the treatment of painful conditions.

Amethocaine eye drops, 1 per cent, are very effective and have a more prolonged effect than cocaine.

Antiseptic eye drops and ointments

These are used in the treatment of various types of conjunctivitis and corneal ulceration. Silver preparations have been employed in the prophylaxis and treatment of ophthalmia neonatorum.

Silver protein (*Guttae argentoproteini mitis*, Argyrol drops).

Zinc sulphate, 0·25 per cent (*Guttae zinci sulphatis*).

Streptomycin.

Sulphacetamide, 'Albucid', 10 per cent (*Guttae sulphacetamidi* and 6% *Oculent. sulphacetamidi.*)

Chloramphenicol ('Chloromycetin') eye drops and ointments.

Castor oil is sometimes instilled into the conjunctiva in cases of corneal abrasion. It is also used after anaesthesia with chloroform or ether, to prevent subsequent inflammation due to the irritation of their vapour.

Flourescein (*Guttae fluoresceini*, 2 per cent), placed in the conjunctival sac, stains corneal abrasions and ulcers and makes them clearly visible.

Hydrocortisone is used in drops (1 per cent) or ointment (2·5 per cent) in allergic conjunctivitis.

Prednisolone (0·5 per cent) eye drops are used for the same purpose.

DRUGS USED IN THE TREATMENT OF SYPHILIS

Syphilis is a disease caused by the *Spirochaeta pallida* (*Treponema pallidum*). Its clinical manifestations occur in three stages:

1. The primary sore or chancre.

2. The secondary stage, commencing about 6 weeks after infection and lasting up to 2 years, during which skin rashes and various other symptoms may arise.

3. The tertiary stage in which gummata are found. The cardiovascular system, bones or nervous system may be affected.

Congenital syphilis may also occur.

The routine treatment of syphilis is to give a full course of penicillin (e.g. 600,000 units of procaine penicillin daily for ten days) or one of the other antibiotics (tetracyclines or erythromycin). Further treatment is controlled by the results of the Wasserman reaction. In some cases of tertiary syphilis a course of bismuth injections may be given before penicillin is commenced. Arsenic and mercury preparations are no longer employed.

METALLIC DRUGS

I. Arsenic

Acetarsol vaginal tablets (SVC) contain organic arsenic compounds and they are used in cases of vaginal discharge (leucorrhoea), especially that due to infection with *Trichomonas vaginalis*.

Poisoning by inorganic arsenic

This may be suicidal or homicidal. Arsenic is present in many weed-killers, in which form it is most easily obtained. The symptoms depend on the dosage taken. A large dose produces epigastric pain, vomiting, diarrhoea, excessive thirst, muscular cramps and collapse which may soon terminate fatally. Smaller doses given over a longer period result in loss of appetite, intermittent attacks of diarrhoea, thirst, colicky abdominal pains, pigmentation of the skin and symptoms of peripheral neuritis such as wrist-drop, numbness and loss of tendon reflexes. Arsenic remains in the body for some time and can be recovered from the hair, nails, liver and other organs.

II. Mercury (*Hydrargyrum*)

Mercury or quicksilver (having the chemical symbol of Hg) is an element which has the form of a bright liquid metal. It is used in thermometers, and also in the sphygmomanometer and other types of pressure gauge. The metal itself is an ingredient of a number of preparations used in medicine. Mercury salts are also employed. Mersalyl and 'Neptal', are organic compounds of mercury. Mercury preparations have a number of actions on the body.

(1) *External application*

(*a*) *Antiseptic.* Mercuric chloride (*Hydrargyri perchloridum*, corrosive sublimate) and mercury biniodide are used as antiseptics (p. 38). Mercurochrome and thiomersal ('Merthiolate') are organic mercurial compounds used for external application in the form of solutions, paints, ointments, etc.

H

(*b*) *Antiseptic and antiparasitic ointments.* There are a number of ointments containing mercury used, for example, in the treatment of impetigo and pediculosis pubis, e.g. ammoniated mercury ointment.

Oxide of mercury eye ointment, Golden eye ointment (*oculentum hydrargyri oxidi flavum*) is sometimes used for conjunctivitis and blepharitis.

Some people show special skin sensitivity to mercury, and its application in any form may be followed by a rash.

(2) *Internal administration*

(*a*) *On the alimentary tract.* With large doses the flow of saliva is increased and, if taken over a long period, the mouth and gums become inflamed (stomatitis). Irritation of the intestine is also caused and it will be recalled that calomel has been used as a purgative.

(*b*) *On the kidneys.* Certain mercury preparations, especially mersalyl, are diuretics and increase the flow of urine.

Mercurial poisoning

The acute symptoms include stomatitis, with a metallic taste in the mouth, gastro-enteritis (diarrhoea and vomiting), and nephritis (blood and albumin in the urine), followed by collapse in serious cases. In chronic cases, in addition to any of the above, peripheral neuritis may develop.

III. Bismuth (*Bismuthum*)

Bismuth is employed therapeutically both in its metallic state and in the form of various salts.

Metallic bismuth. Prepared in the form of finely divided particles, may be given by the intramuscular injection of a suspension in glucose solution (*Injectio bismuthi,* 1 ml.), in the treatment of syphilis.

Bismuth salts by mouth have no effect in the treatment of syphilis but are used for various other purposes.

External application

Bismuth subgallate ('Dermatol') This is sometimes used as a dusting powder and ointment in skin conditions.

Bismuth and iodoform paste (BIPP), p. 44.

Internal administration

Bismuth carbonate (*Bismuthi carbonas,* bismuth oxycarbonate), 2 gram (10 to 30 grains), is sometimes used as a weak antacid and gastric sedative in cases of gastritis and gastric ulcer. It is also used in diarrhoea.

DRUGS USED IN THE TREATMENT OF MALARIA

Malaria is essentially a disease acquired in the tropics and caused by the malarial parasite which is introduced into the body by the bite of an infected *Anopheles* mosquito.

The parasite reaches the liver where it develops and divides into many small offspring known as merozoites. These escape into the blood stream and invade the red corpuscles. In these cells they undergo a phase of development and division known as schizogony. The resulting new generation of merozoites is liberated from the red cells into the blood stream. They circulate until each again enters a red corpuscle and the cycle is repeated. Circulating parasites can be destroyed by certain drugs and, in the case of malignant tertian malaria, this is the end of the infection. In all other types of malaria, however, the parasites have a persistent phase in the liver. This is known as the exo-erythrocytic phase and accounts for relapses after successful treatment of acute attacks of malaria. Different drugs are required to destroy the parasites in the liver.

The characteristic feature of the disease is the occurrence of rigors at regular intervals of 48 to 72 hours, according to the species of parasite present. The occurrence of rigors coincides with a fresh generation of young parasites being liberated from the red corpuscles.

Anti-malarial drugs

For many years quinine was the only drug used in the prevention and treatment of malaria. It has now been largely replaced by various synthetic products, e.g.

Proguanil ('Paludrine')
Chloroquine (e.g. 'Nivaquine')
Primaquine
Pyrimethamine ('Daraprim')

Anti-malarial drugs may be given:

(a) *Prophylactically*

It is a usual practice for persons living in malaria-infested districts to take regular doses of an anti-malarial drug in order to suppress or prevent the disease if they happen to be bitten by an infected mosquito.

Those generally used are:

Proguanil 100–300 mg daily.

Pyrimethamine 25–50 mg once weekly.

Chloroquine preparations in weekly doses of 300 mg of the base.

Amodiaquine in weekly doses of 400 mg of the base.

(b) *For the treatment of an attack*

Chloroquine preparations, 600 mg of the base followed by 300 mg 6 hours later and then 300 mg daily for two days or amodiaquine

600 mg base for the first 24 hours, then 400 mg daily for 2 more days.

In cerebral malaria and other serious types chloroquine may be given by intramuscular injection or by intravenous drip. Quinine can also be given intravenously but intramuscular injection is likely to cause abscess formation.

(c) *For the treatment of the residual infection in the liver*

As explained earlier, infection persists in the liver in all types of malaria excepting the malignant tertian variety. **Primaquine** is used to eradicate the liver infection. It is given orally in a dose of 7·5 mg of the base twice daily for 14 days. It may be given concurrently with or following the treatment of the acute attack with chloroquine, amodiaquine or quinine.

Primaquine may cause cyanosis, nausea, vomiting, diarrhoea and abdominal pain. Haemolysis may occur in the blood vessels resulting in anaemia. This complication is more common in some dark-skinned races, owing to an inherited enzyme deficiency. Patients under treatment with primaquine should be under observation for toxic effects. Pamaquine is more toxic than primaquine and has fallen into disfavour.

Mepacrine ('Atebrin')

This was the first synthetic anti-malarial drug and was of great value during the Second World War. It is slow in action, however, and stains the skin yellow. It occasionally causes mental disturbances. Its use in malaria is no longer recommended where other drugs are available. The drug is still of value in the treatment of tapeworm infestation.

N.B.—The real prophylaxis of malaria is to destroy the breeding grounds of the mosquito by draining stagnant water or preventing the hatching of the larva into the adult mosquito by covering such pools with paraffin. A bed net to prevent bites at night is also essential.

Quinine (*Quinina*)

Quinine is an alkaloid obtained from cinchona bark which is cultivated in the East Indies, India and Ceylon In addition to its now very limited use in malaria it is also employed occasionally for other purposes in therapeutics.

Other uses of quinine

1. *Antipyretic*. Quinine has an antipyretic action and is occasionally used

in the treatment of coryza and mild febrile illnesses. Ammoniated tincture of quinine is a favourite preparation.

2. As a *bitter*. Quinine has a bitter flavour and helps to improve the appetite. It is therefore sometimes included in tonics.

3. In *obstetrics*. Its former use for the medical induction of labour has been mentioned (p. 213).

4. In *surgery*. Quinine and urethane solutions have been used for the injection of varicose veins.

Quinine and urea hydrochloride, 1 per cent, may be injected to produce local relief from pain in fibrositis, lumbago, etc.

5. To prevent *muscle cramps* at night, 300–600 mg (5–10 gr.) of any of the quinine salts may be taken before retiring. In *myotonia*, a condition where the patient finds it difficult to relax his grip (for example), the dose is 300 mg t.d.s. Procainamide is more effective in this condition.

Some preparations of quinine

Quinine sulphate (*Quininae sulphas*). This is also contained in ammoniated tincture or solution of quinine and in various quinine mixtures.

Quinine bisulphate. **Quinine dihydrochloride.**

Quinine poisoning and idiosyncrasy, see p. 27.

Quinidine (p. 88) is another alkaloid obtained from cinchona and is used to prevent the recurrence of cardiac dyshythmias (e.g. atrial fibrilation) after D.C. cardioversion.

DRUGS USED IN THE TREATMENT OF RHEUMATOID ARTHRITIS

Gold salts

Gold salts are used in therapeutics in the treatment of rheumatoid arthritis.

The first gold preparation to be employed was 'Sanocrysin' (gold sodium thiosulphate), for the treatment of pulmonary tuberculosis. The exact mode of action of gold salts in rheumatoid arthritis is uncertain.

A number of preparations are available, and are given by intramuscular injection. The one usually employed is injection of sodium aurothiomalate ('Myocrisin').

Dosage. The dosage varies according to the case. As a rule small doses at weekly intervals, commencing with 10 mg, increasing gradually up to 100 mg are the maximum employed. Courses, therefore, last for some weeks, and after an interval of 2 months may be repeated.

Toxic effects

Gold, when injected, has a cumulative effect owing to its slow excretion. Important toxic results may be observed, especially in some persons who show special idiosyncrasy and when large doses are used. They include:

Skin eruptions.   Stomatitis.   Diarrhoea.

Blood disorders, including agranulocytosis and purpura.

Albuminuria. It is wise to test the urine of all patients receiving gold at regular intervals.

It is also necessary to avoid exposure to direct sunlight by sunbathing and also ultra-violet light while gold is being given, because permanent pigmentation of the skin may follow. Dimercaprol (BAL) is used in the treatment of overdosage.

Other anti-rheumatic drugs

Other drugs used in the treatment of rheumatoid arthritis are aspirin, phenylbutazone, ibuprofen, indomethacin, corticosteroids and chloroquine.

Indomethacin ('Indocid') is an anti-inflammatory analgesic which is given by mouth or in suppositories. The oral dose varies between 25 mg twice daily and 50 mg four times a day. There are many possible adverse reactions including peptic ulceration, oedema and purpura.

Ibuprofen ('Brufen') is a rather weaker anti-inflammatory analgesic but it is usually well tolerated and adverse reactions appear to be neither severe nor frequent. It is given orally in a dose of 200 mg three times a day.

Chloroquine may be beneficial in rheumatoid arthritis but careful supervision by an ophthalmologist is necessary because this drug may damage the eyes (cornea and retina).

ALCOHOL

Alcohol is a substance of wide social usage but it must also be regarded as a potential poison and a drug of addiction. Its use as a therapeutic measure has been steadily decreasing in medical practice although it probably has a limited sphere of usefulness.

Its main pharmacological actions may be summarized thus:

1. It is a central nervous system depressant. The apparent stimulating effect in the first instance is due to abolition of the normal mental control of the higher centres of the brain thereby removing inhibitions and anxiety. Progressively its toxic effects precipitate disturbance of behaviour, inco-ordination of muscular

movements and speech and, finally, coma which may prove fatal.

2. It acts as a peripheral vasodilator which gives rise to a general feeling of warmth. In the stomach this may temporarily improve the appetite.

3. It is readily metabolized into carbon dioxide and water, providing a number of calories. It is, therefore, to some extent of food value especially as it is quickly absorbed from the stomach.

4. Excessive intake has a diuretic action, hence the headache and dry mouth due to dehydration in a "hang-over."

5. Continued intake is liable to cause defective absorption of vitamins, in particular those of the B complex.

The clinical effects of alcohol

Although many people consume moderate quantities of alcoholic liquor without any obvious harmful effect the clinical manifestations of excess may be considered as:

(*a*) acute and (*b*) chronic alcoholism.

Acute alcoholism. The symptoms of progressive drunkenness are too obvious and well known to require further description. Several special points should, however, be remembered.

(*a*) It may precipitate an epileptic fit or migraine in persons subject to these conditions.

(*b*) Alcohol greatly increases the effect of barbiturates, narcotics and some other drugs.

(*c*) It may obscure cerebral or other injury sustained in the inebriated state, sometimes with fatal results.

(*d*) In any case it is unwise to administer it as "first aid" treatment as the odour of the breath may cause the false impression that the individual is drunk rather than suffering from some organic lesion.

Treatment. In the early stages, before unconsciousness, the simplest measure is to induce vomiting by tickling the back of the throat followed by drinking at least a pint of water which may be repeated at intervals. In comatose patients gastric lavage after ensuring that there is no respiratory obstruction and, if necessary, using an endotracheal tube to avoid the inhalation of vomitus. Intravenous glucose, injections of nikethamide and vitamin B may be helpful.

The post-alcoholic syndrome ("hang-over") may be helped by further intake of water or fruit juice sweetened with sugar or glucose and moderate doses of paracetamol or aspirin. The associated anorexia is usually self-limiting. Whether further small doses of alcohol ("the hair of the dog") are helpful is a matter of individual experience.

Chronic alcoholism. While it must be admitted that some individuals consume considerable quantities of alcohol over many years without ever being obviously intoxicated and without it having any obvious adverse effects, in others many serious conditions may develop. These include:

(*a*) Effects on the nervous system, e.g. neuritis, muscular inco-ordination ("the shakes"), progressive mental deterioration (alcoholic dementia), insomnia, hallucinations and delirium tremens.

(*b*) Cirrhosis of the liver and its associated symptoms.

(*c*) Chronic gastritis associated with dyspeptic symptoms, vomiting, anorexia and malnutrition.

(*d*) Vitamin deficiency, particularly B_{12}, which may be associated with optic neuritis and visual defects

(*e*) Degeneration of the heart (alcoholic cardiomyopathy).

Treatment. The management of alcohol dependence is essentially a matter for experts and often requires institutional treatment. Gradual reduction of intake covered by sedative drugs help to minimize withdrawal symptoms. Special drugs such as 'Antabuse' or aversion therapy with apomorphine, given to produce vomiting every time an alcoholic drink is taken, are sometimes employed.

"Alcoholics Anonymous" is a worldwide organization which is of value to the reformed, but once an individual has been weaned from the habit a single drink may restart the addiction.

Medical uses and abuses

It is not always wise to cut off the supply of alcohol from a patient suffering from an acute disease who is accustomed to its use. In some cases of bronchopneumonia and gastro-enteritis in young babies small doses of brandy often induce sleep and act as an easily absorbed foodstuff. A small drink at night sometimes helps the insomnia of the elderly but appropriate sedatives, if necessary, are less expensive!

Its use should be forbidden in cases of infective hepatitis, jaundice and peptic ulcer and when it might potentiate the action of any other drugs which are being taken. On the other hand if it produces a feeling of well-being in the terminal stages of cancer or similar fatal conditions its use is certainly justified.

External uses

It has already been mentioned (p. 38) that alcohol and methylated spirit have antiseptic properties and that they harden the skin. Further, their rapid evaporation makes them a useful basis for cooling lotions in the treatment of sprains and contusions.

The alcohol content of various wines and spirits, etc

Liqueurs	50 per cent
Brandy, whisky, rum, gin . . .	40 per cent
Port and sherry	20 per cent
Burgundy	up to 14 per cent
Champagne, claret, hock . . .	10 per cent
Beer and stout	2 to 5 per cent

Disulfiram ('Antabuse')

Disulfiram is used, together with psychiatric treatment, to treat chronic alcoholics. It interferes with the metabolism of alcohol, causing aldehyde to accumulate in the body. This causes nausea and vomiting, severe flushing, throbbing headache, palpitations and dyspnoea.

The resulting discomfort discourages the patient from drinking alcohol.

When large quantities of alcohol are consumed the reaction may be severe, with hypotension and collapse. Such a reaction is treated with oxygen, intravenous dextrose and, perhaps, antihistamines.

The following dosage is used for disulfiram:

Day 1 800 mg	Day 4 200 mg
Day 2 600 mg	Day 5 200 mg
Day 3 400 mg	

Subsequently 100–200 mg daily for up to one year i.e. $\frac{1}{2}$ to 1 tablet.

CHAPTER 17

The Sulphonamide Drugs

For many years chemists and physicians have been working to produce chemical substances which would influence bacterial disease. An early outcome was the preparation of the arsenical compounds for use in the treatment of syphilis. Later it was found that certain complicated chemical compounds of the sulphonamide type, of which 'Prontosil' or sulphanilamide was the first, were effective in the treatment of streptococcal infections. This led to the preparation of numerous other compounds of the same kind and their employment in other varieties of bacterial disease. Some years later the antibiotics were discovered.

Although sulphonamides have been superseded by antibiotics in the treatment of many diseases, they still play a part in the management of some types of meningitis, bacillary dysentery and infections of the urinary tract.

They may also be useful against organisms which have become resistant to antibiotics but have remained sensitive to sulphonamides, or may be given to patients who have developed sensitivity reactions to antibiotics.

Mode of action

Sulphonamides do not actually kill bacteria but prevent their growth and multiplication in the body so that the natural immunity of the individual can exterminate the infection. They act by preventing bacteria from using para-amino-benzoic acid, a substance necessary in their metabolism. They are, therefore, bacteriostatic in action. The main principle in their administration is to produce rapidly a high concentration of the substance in the blood and to maintain this concentration for some days, until pyrexia and symptoms due to the disease have subsided. In order to reduce the risk of the patient developing drug sensitivity or agranulocytosis their administration should not usually be continued for more than ten days.

With the exception of the meningococcus, which is very rarely resistant, most other organisms which are initially sensitive to sulphonamides may become resistant. Sensitivity tests are, therefore, important.

THE SULPHONAMIDES

The widespread use and manufacture of these drugs has resulted in a multiplicity of preparations and names. According to their practical use they fall into four main groups:

1. Sulphonamides used for general infections.
2. Sulphonamides used for urinary infections.
3. Sulphonamides used for intestinal infections.
4. Sulphonamides for local use.

Those used for general infections may also be employed for the other purposes mentioned.

1. Sulphonamides for general infections

The most important is: sulphadimidine ('Sulphamezathine').

Others include:

Sulphathiazole   Sulphadiazine   Sulphafurazole ('Gantrisin') Trisulphonamide ('Sulphatriad'), a mixture of sulphadiazine, sulphathiazole and sulphamerazine.

Long-acting sulphonamides. These include: sulphamethoxypyridazine ('Midicel', 'Lederkyn'). One dose (0·5–1 G) is sufficient for 24 hours. For prevention of streptococcal sore throats and recurrences of rheumatic fever, the drug need be given only once a week. Sulphaphenazole ('Orisulf') is given in doses of 500 mg twice daily.

Among the conditions in which sulphonamide therapy has been used with success are:

Streptococcal infections. Infection by the streptococcus may produce many different manifestations of disease. In most instances, however, penicillin or one of the other antibiotics will be the drug of choice.

The following are common conditions due to streptococcal infection: puerperal sepsis, erysipelas, tonsillitis, cellutitis, otitis media, acute mastoiditis and streptococcal meningitis.

Scarlet fever is also due to a streptococcus, but sulphonamides have not proved effective in the acute disease, although they are of some value in the treatment of certain complications, such as otitis media.

Meningococcal infections. Sulphadimidine and sulphadiazine are often effective in the treatment of meningococcal meningitis, but meningococci may become resistant to the drug.

Gonococcal infections. Sulphonamides have been employed in the treatment of gonorrhoea both in the acute and chronic stages, but one of the antibiotics is usually employed.

Pneumococcal infections. Not every case of pneumonia responds and usually penicillin or one of the other antibiotics is employed.

2. Sulphonamides for urinary infections

In addition to the sulphonamides mentioned above for use in general infections, the following are highly soluble and are particularly active against the *Escherichia coli*. They are, therefore, employed in cases of pyelitis and cystitis p. 129:

Sulphamethizole ('Urolucosil', 100–200 mg)

Nitrofurantoin ('Furadantin'), 100 mg, six hourly, is not a sulphonamide but is used as a urinary antiseptic.

3. Sulphonamides for intestinal infections

All the sulphonamides previously mentioned are soluble and are, therefore, easily absorbed into the blood stream from the alimentary tract. There are a number of insoluble sulphonamides which are not absorbed and therefore continue to act on bacteria throughout the whole length of the bowel. These drugs include:

Sulphaguanidine

Phthalylsulphathiazole ('Sulfathalidine')

Succinylsulphathiazole ('Sulfasuxidine', 'Cremosuxidine')

They are used for intestinal infections, e.g. bacillary dysentery. Some doctors prefer the absorbable sulphonamides, however, believing that tissue levels of sulphonamide are more important than the quantity of the drug in the lumen of the bowel.

Unfortunately, most dysentery organisms are now resistant to sulphonamides. Antibiotic (e.g. neomycin) therapy is therefore usually preferable, but sulphonamides may be useful in prophylaxis. Sulphaguanidine is suitable for this purpose, since no systemic effect is required.

Salicylazosulphapyridine ('Salazopyrin') is a sulphonamide used in the treatment of ulcerative colitis.

4. Sulphonamides for local use

Sulphonamides have been applied to the skin in the form of ointments in the treatment of various skin diseases, but they may cause sensitization and dermatitis and are, therefore, now avoided.

Sulphacetamide eye drops and eye ointment are however, very useful in the treatment of infections of the conjunctiva.

Methods of administration

In the majority of cases the drugs are given by mouth but, to gravely ill patients and those who vomit excessively, sodium salt preparations may be administered by intramuscular injection or intravenously. They may be conveniently given by the latter method when the patient is receiving saline by the continuous intravenous drip technique by injecting the required dose at regular intervals through the rubber tubing leading to the vein.

Dosage

When given for general infections the dosage of the soluble sulphonamides must be carefully adjusted to the age of the patient. It is usual to commence with a single large dose (double that which is subsequently given) in order to ensure a rapid high concentration of the drug in the blood. Tablets of the drug (each of which usually contains 0·5 gram) are given by mouth and may be chewed or powdered and swallowed with a glass of water. An alternative and better method is to crush and suspend in milk, glucose–saline or a mucilage of tragacanth. If the drug is not tolerated by mouth, special preparations for intramuscular injection may be used. It must be emphasized, however, that deep intramuscular injections must be given into the buttock. Subcutaneous injection leads to the gradual formation of a painful abscess, leaving an ulcer which takes a long time to heal.

The usual initial adult dose is 2 grams, followed by 1 gram six-hourly. (Sulphadiazine is given every 6 to 8 hours and 'Sulphamerazine' every 8 to 12 hours.) The administration of the drug is generally continued for a day or two after the temperature has fallen to normal, as premature withdrawal is often followed by recurrence of pyrexia and the infective process.

Toxic effects

The toxic effects are mainly allergic and include headache, nausea and vomiting. Occasionally skin rashes, polyarteritis, Stevens–

Johnson syndrome and agranulocytosis occur. Unless sufficient fluid is given at the same time some of the earlier sulphonamides tend to crystallize in the urine causing haematuria and even suppression of urine. This is particularly likely to occur if dehydration is present as a result of diarrhoea or excessive sweating. In these circumstances an adequate fluid intake must be maintained and it is advisable to render the urine alkaline with potassium citrate.

'Septrin' and 'Bactrim'. These antibacterial drugs consist of a mixture of trimethoprim and sulphamethoxazole and are superior to sulphonamides and some antibiotics in their bactericidal action. They are effective in the treatment of bronchitis, gonorrhoea and most urinary infections and have been used with success in brucellosis, typhoid fever and infections caused by other bacteria of the salmonella group. Tablets and paediatric preparations are available but the drug should be avoided during pregnancy and in individuals who are sulphonamide-sensitive.

CHAPTER 18

Antibiotics

An antibiotic is a chemical substance produced by micro-organisms or moulds which prevents the growth (bacteriostatic) of or kills (bactericidal) other micro-organisms.

The most important are:

The Penicillins.

The Cephalosporins e.g. cephaloridine ('Ceporin').

The Tetracyclines

    (a) Tetracycline ('Tetracyn').

    (b) Chlortetracycline ('Aureomycin').

    (c) Oxytetracycline ('Terramycin').

    (d) The newer tetracyclines.

Erythromycin, Spiramycin, Oleandomycin.

Novobiocin.

Chloramphenicol ('Chloromycetin').

Fusidic acid ('Fucidin').

Polymyxin B and Colistin ('Colomycin').

Bacitracin.

Nystatin, Griseofulvin, Amphotericin B.

Streptomycin, Viomycin.

Each antibiotic has its own sphere of activity against the common bacteria. Some ("broad-spectrum" antibiotics) are effective against a wide range of organisms, to others only a few are sensitive, but fortunately most of the common organisms are affected by at least one of the antibiotics. On the other hand, the only "viruses" which are sensitive are those causing lympho-granuloma venereum and psittacosis, which are sensitive to the tetracycline group. Unfortunately, the other more common viruses, causing poliomyelitis, measles, mumps, chicken pox and small pox are uninfluenced by any of the present known antibiotics. The organism (*Mycoplasma*) causing primary atypical pneumonia (form-erly regarded as a virus pneumonia) is sensitive to tetracyclines.

Disadvantages

1. Bacterial resistance

As with sulphonamides, an important drawback to the use of antibiotics is that many bacteria acquire resistance to them after a period of treatment and continue to breed resistant organisms which can cause further disease. This will no longer respond to treatment with the same antibiotic. For example, the tubercle bacillus quickly develops resistance to streptomycin. Staphylococci also acquire resistance both to penicillin and drugs of the tetracycline group.

2. Toxic effects and hypersensitivity

Gastro-intestinal irritation, nausea, vomiting and diarrhoea may occur when antibiotics are given by mouth.

Skin sensitivity may develop to penicillin or streptomycin causing rashes, not only in patients but also in nurses and others handling the drug. Streptomycin may have a serious toxic effect on the vestibular and auditory nerve causing vertigo and deafness.

Very rarely anaphylactic shock with collapse and even death may follow the administration of penicillin in hypersensitive individuals.

For future reference, it is wise to make a conspicuous note on a patient's record if *any* drug sensitivity is observed and the individual should be warned.

3. Super-infection

This applies especially to the antibiotics given by mouth which by killing off some of the normal bacteria inhabiting the alimentary canal permit the overgrowth of other insensitive ones which can cause serious complications.

In particular, there may be an overgrowth of yeasts and fungi (usually *Candida albicans*, the fungus causing thrush) which cause soreness of the mouth and anal regions, or which may even extend into the bronchi and lungs with fatal results.

Staphylococci may develop resistance to penicillin and the tetracyclines and cause serious gastro-enteritis or other infections. Such resistant staphylococci are likely to be susceptible to erythromycin, methicillin, cloxacillin, flucloxacillin, fusidic acid, cephaloridine, cephalexin, novobiocin, neomycin, vancomycin, or chloramphenicol.

4. Alterations in vitamin formation and absorption from the bowel

The Vitamin B complex, including riboflavin and nicotinic acid, is particularly affected, so that this is sometimes given at the same time as an oral antiobiotic, although this is probably only necessary if the administration is prolonged beyond five days and in debilitated patients.

5. Aplastic anaemia

Chloramphenicol may occasionally produce aplastic anaemia or agranulocytosis.

THE PENICILLINS

These consist of
1. Natural penicillins (G and V).
2. Semisynthetic penicillins.

Benzylpenicillin (Penicillin G)

This substance, which was the first antibiotic to be used, and is often simply referred to as "penicillin", is the active principle of a mould (*Penicillium notatum*) which has a marked action on many bacteria. In the usual doses it is bactericidal. In many instances it is more effective than the sulphonamide drugs and has practically no toxic effects except in sensitive individuals. Although it has a moderately wide range of action not all bacteria are affected by it and even some of those which are can eventually develop some degree of resistance to it.

It is usually given by intramuscular injection but may be given orally, intravenously and intrathecally (in small doses only.)

Indications

The suitability of a case for treatment with penicillin depends not so much on the nature of the disease as on the susceptibility of the micro-organism causing it: some species are highly susceptible and others far too resistant for this treatment to have any effect. It follows that in diseases which may be caused by any of several different bacteria (e.g. meningitis, peritonitis) a bacteriological diagnosis and sensitivity test is usually necessary if treatment is to be undertaken with any assurance of success.

The chief organisms susceptible to benzylpenicillin are:

H*

Gonococcus	Diphtheria bacillus
Meningococcus	Organisms of gas gangrene
Streptococcus	Spirochaetes of syphilis and of Weil's disease
Staphylococcus	Actinomyces
Pneumococcus	Anthrax bacillus

Diseases in which penicillin may be used—examples are:

septicaemia	actinomycosis	carbuncles
puerperal sepsis	anthrax	suppurative arthritis
cellulitis	gonorrhoea	bacterial endocarditis
osteomyelitis	gas gangrene	syphilis
pneumonia	meningitis	

Penicillin is of no value in the following conditions for which it should *not* be used except when some intercurrent infection is present:

Tuberculosis

Ulcerative colitis

Infections caused by viruses such as influenza, poliomyelitis and encephalitis.

All Gram–negative bacillary infections such as whooping cough, typhoid fever, dysentery, undulant fever, and infections with *Escherichia coli*.

Properties of penicillin

(*a*) Once penicillin has been removed from the ampoule or vial it is likely to deteriorate, particularly if exposed to moisture or heat. Solutions or other preparations of penicillin exposed to air and kept at room temperature will not deteriorate significantly in 24 hours, but should be kept in a refrigerator.

(*b*) Penicillin passes rapidly from the blood into the tissues, but the serous membranes and meninges present a barrier which penicillin does not readily penetrate. Hence intrathecal and intrapleural injections may be necessary.

(*c*) Penicillin is rapidly excreted; for this reason it must be given in sufficient dosage to maintain an adequate concentration in the blood. Blood concentrations may be raised by blocking renal excretion of penicillin with probenecid 500 mg 6-hourly.

(*d*) The diffusion of penicillin into dead tissues is slow; sequestra, large sloughs, or collections of pus, are, therefore, likely to harbour bacteria out of reach of the drug, and these usually have to be removed if treatment is to be effective.

Types of benzylpenicillin

Penicillin is an acid substance which forms salts with sodium, potassium and calcium and can be combined with other substances.

There are therefore several different forms of benzylpenicillin which differ somewhat from each other and are used for special purposes.

1. **Plain benzylpenicillin** or **soluble penicillin** (known also as crystalline penicillin G) which is commonly employed for repeated intramuscular injections in doses of 500,000 to 1 million units (1 mega unit) every 4–12 hours, according to the severity of the infection. 'Falapen' is a form of benzylpenicillin which may be administered orally in twice daily doses of 500,000 units, preferably before a meal.

2. **Procaine penicillin,** sometimes prescribed as 'Distaquaine,' which is less soluble and therefore more slowly absorbed. It is given in doses of 300,000–600,000 units daily by intramuscular injection. In order to get a more rapid effect the first injection may be combined with a similar dose of soluble benzylpenicillin. In gonorrhoea, one injection of procaine penicillin, 600,000 units is adequate if the organism is sensitive to pencillin but there are now resistant strains.

3. **Benzathine penicillin** ('Penidural') is even less soluble and more slowly absorbed. A single intramuscular injection of 600,000–1 million units may give an effective blood level lasting several days. A hard lump may develop at the site of injection.

4. Combinations of the various types of penicillin are available. Oily preparations which delay absorption are sometimes used in syphilis (e.g. Procaine penicillin in oil with aluminium monostearate, PAM) and there are other preparations in which penicillin is mixed with streptomycin (e.g. 'Crystamycin') or sulphonamides.

N.B.—Penicillin is not administered at the same time as tetracycline because the bactericidal effect of the former is diminished by the bacterostatic action of the latter.

Modes of administration

Benzylpenicillin may be administered in the following ways:

1. *Intramuscular injection.*

2. *Intravenous solution. Soluble* penicillin may be injected intravenously in doses similar to those given by intramuscular injection depending on the nature and severity of the infection.

3. *Intrathecal injection* may be used in certain cases of meningitis. Only specially prepared *soluble* penicillin well diluted, should be employment. One dose of 20,000 units in twenty-four hours is sufficient and 30,000 units should not be exceeded.

4. *Intrapleural injection* may be used in the treatment of empyema.

5. *Local application.* Penicillin has been used in the form of a solution, a cream and a powder. In the latter instance it has been mixed with a sulphonamide and blown with an insufflator onto raw surfaces or into wounds twice daily.

Apart from eye drops, local applications are inadvisable and should be discouraged on account of the liability of producing a sensitization rash which may be worse than the original condition.

6. *Orally,* as in the prophylaxis of recurrences of rheumatic fever.

The duration of treatment varies considerably according to the condition and response of the patient, but should seldom be for less than 5 days or more than 12 days. Treatment is usually continued for about 2 days after a favourable response has been obtained. If no response is obtained within 72 hours another antibiotic will probably be needed.

Toxic reactions. Penicillin is usually non-toxic, but it occasionally gives rise to delayed reactions, such as fever, and urticarial rashes. These may be treated with antihistamine drugs and the local application of calamine lotion.

Rarely, as previously mentioned, an immediate reaction—*anaphylactic shock*—with collapse and even death may occur. In this type of reaction adrenaline 1 ml. (1 in 1000) should be injected subcutaneously at once, followed by intravenous hydrocortisone (100 mg) and an intravenous antihistamine (e.g. chlorpheniramine ('Piriton') 10 mg. Before giving penicillin, it is wise routinely to enquire about previous sensitivity and also if the patient is subject to asthma or other allergic conditions.

Phenoxymethylpenicillin (Penicillin V)

Unlike benzylpenicillin, this is able to resist inactivation by gastric hydrochloric acid. It is therefore used as an oral penicillin. Dose: 125 to 250 mg every 4 hours.

The semisynthetic penicillins

These are produced by the addition of side-chains to the penicillin nucleus, which was isolated in 1959. They may be classified into three types, examples of which are shown in the following table.

TABLE 6.—THE SEMISYNTHETIC PENICILLINS

Acid-resistant	Penicillinase-resistant	Broad-spectrum
Phenethicillin ('Broxil') Propicillin ('Brocillin')	Methicillin ('Celbenin' Cloxacillin ('Orbenin') Flucloxacillin ('Floxapen')	Ampicillin ('Penbritin') Carbenicillin ('Pyopen')

The acid-resistant penicillins

These resist inactivation by gastric hydrochloric acid and are, therefore, used as oral penicillins. Phenoxymethylpenicillin and phenethicillin are highly satisfactory and are given in a dosage of 125–250 mg 4–6 hourly. They are generally indicated in minor infections (e.g. acute tonsillitis) by highly susceptible organisms (e.g. haemolytic streptococci).

The penicillinase-resistant penicillins

Benzylpenicillin is inactivated by the enzyme penicillinase, which some bacteria (e.g. resistant staphylococci) produce. Some of the semisynthetic penicillins are resistant to staphylococcal penicillinase and are therefore used against benzylpenicillin-resistant staphylococci. Methicillin ('Celbenin') is inactivated by gastric acid and must, therefore, be given parenterally. The dose is 1 G intramuscularly every 4 to 6 hours. Cloxacillin ('Orbenin') can be given orally, 500 mg 6 hourly, or intramuscularly, 250 mg 4–6 hourly. Flucloxacillin ('Floxapen') is absorbed more readily and the usual dose by mouth is 250 mg 6 hourly.

Broad-spectrum penicillins

Ampicillin ('Penbritin') is the one used widely. It is active against a wide range of bacteria, including strains of *E. coli*, *Salmonella*, *Shigella*, *H. influenzae*, *Proteus mirabilis* (but not other *Proteus* species) and enterococci. Of particular value is the activity against Gram-negative bacilli, an activity which benzylpenicillin lacks. It is used principally in urinary tract infections (500 mg 8 hourly) and in chronic bronchitis (usually 250 mg but up to 1 G 6 hourly). Ampicillin may also be used in the treatment of sub-acute bacterial endocarditis, the serum level of the drug being increased by concomitant administration of probenecid. Ampicillin is effective, at a dose of 8 G *per diem*, in typhoid fever but chloramphenicol is more rapid in action and is the treatment of choice. Ampicillin is excreted in urine and bile and, because of the high concentration reached in the latter secretion, it is useful in the treatment of typhoid carriers.

GENERAL POINTS ABOUT THE PENICILLINS

1. Benzylpenicillin remains the penicillin of choice for pneumococcal pneumonia and many other conditions.

2. Hypersensitive patients show cross-reactivity to all the penicillins.

3. Oral penicillins are best given on an empty stomach (or $\frac{1}{2}$ hour a.c.) in order to promote absorption and hence achieve high serum levels.

THE CEPHALOSPORINS

These are derivatives of a fungus isolated from the sea near a sewage outfall in Sardinia. One (Cephalosporin N) is a broad-spectrum penicillin (otherwise known as Penicillin N). Cephalosporin C has a nucleus similar to that of penicillin.

Cephaloridine ('Ceporin') is a semisynthetic cephalosporin made by adding a side-chain to the nucleus of Cephalosporin C. It is highly bactericidal, especially against Gram-negative organisms. It is a broad-spectrum antibiotic having an even wider range of antibacterial activity than ampicillin Being excreted unchanged in the urine, high urinary levels of the antibiotic are reached. It is of value in the treatment of acute pyelonephritis. There seems to be a remarkable lack of toxicity and it is therefore a suitable drug to use against Gram-negative infections in anuric patients. Other drugs easily reach toxic levels in the sera of these patients.

This antibiotic is poorly absorbed from the gastrointestinal tract and it must, therefore, be given by injection (intramuscularly or intravenously).

Cephalexin ('Ceporex', 'Keflex')

Cephalosporins are now available which are readily absorbed from the gastrointestinal tract and are therefore administered orally. Cephalexin is one of these and is usually given in a dose of 250–500 mg six-hourly. Up to 1 G six-hourly may be prescribed for pneumonias, however. One of its many uses is before and after dental surgery in a patient with rheumatic heart disease who is regularly taking penicillin to prevent recurrences of acute rheumatism. The organisms which might cause subacute bacterial endocarditis, in such a patient, may be resistant to penicillin, to which they have become "acclimatized".

In brief, the cephalosporins have a broad spectrum of activity, low toxicity and little tendency to cause allergic reactions. They are used orally for the treatment of genito-urinary and respiratory tract infections and by intramuscular injection for the prevention of bacterial endocarditis. They are used intravenously for bacteraemias and septicaemias.

It should be noted that cephalexin may cause a false positive reaction for glucose in the urine with Benedict's or Fehling's solutions, or with 'Clinitest' tablets, but not with enzyme tests such as 'Clinistix.'

Chloramphenicol ('Chloromycetin')

This is a crystalline substance originally obtained from the mould *Streptomyces Venezuelae* and which can also be prepared synthetically. It is bacteriostatic.

It may be indicated in:

1. Typhoid fever.

2. *Haemophilus* meningitis and *Klebsiella pneumoniae* infections.

3. Life-threatening infections in which other antibiotics will not suffice.

Some individuals, especially children, are sensitive to chloramphenicol and the drug may affect the bone marrow causing *aplastic anaemia* or agranulocytosis which may prove fatal. It may occur after relatively small doses. The danger to adults is very small provided the course of treatment does not exceed ten days.

It is supplied in capsules each containing 250 mg. It has a bitter taste which is sometimes a disadvantage when given to children unless concealed in honey or given in the form of a special preparation ('Chloromycetin palmitate').

The dose is 250 to 500 mg every four or six hours.

Ointments are available, also eye drops and ear drops. These local applications are free from the danger of producing blood dyscrasias.

THE TETRACYCLINES

These include:

(a) **Tetracycline** ('Tetracyn', 'Achromycin').

(b) **Chlortetracycline** (Aureomycin').

(c) **Oxytetracycline** ('Terramycin').

(d) The newer tetracyclines, e.g. demethylchlortetracycline ('Ledermycin') methacycline ('Rondomycin') lymecycline ('Tetralysal').

Although 'Aureomycin' and 'Terramycin' were the first drugs of this group to be isolated and used, chemically they are both derived from a substance tetracycline which also has antibiotic effects similar to the others.

'Aureomycin' and 'Terramycin' differ slightly in chemical composition but have a very similar antibiotic range which covers not only those organisms which are generally sensitive to penicillin but also an agent (*Mycoplasma*) causing primary atypical ("virus") pneumonia, rickettsiae, coxiclla (Q fever) and some of the larger "viruses" (Psittacosis). They are sometimes useful against staphylococci which are resistant to penicillin, but staphylococci and streptococci can also develop resistance against tetracyclines. They may be used in chronic bronchitis, where infective episodes are often due to the influenza bacillus (*Haemophilus influenzae*) and the pneumococcus (*Streptococcus pneumoniae*). They are of value in the treatment of diverticulitis of the colon.

The first three tetracyclines are usually given by mouth in doses of 500 mg followed by 250 mg every 4 to 6 hours for five days.

Special preparations are available for intravenous and intramuscular injections and local applications such as drops and ointments are also in use.

The physicochemical properties of lymecycline make it eminently suitable for intramuscular or intravenous use. Otherwise, there seems little reason to prefer the new tetracyclines to the old. All of the tetracyclines have the same antibacterial spectrum.

Tetracyclines given during pregnancy and the first few years of life may cause permanent discoloration of the developing teeth.

Erythromycin (200–500 mg, 6 hourly)

This is an antibiotic having a similar range of action to penicillin. It is used against staphylococci which have become resistant to other antibiotics. Resistance to erythromycin also develops rapidly so that its use against staphylococci should be restricted to selected and urgent cases. One of its principal uses now is in situations where penicillin is indicated but cannot be given because of the patient's hypersensitivity. Proprietary preparations include 'Erythrocin' and 'Ilotycin'. Intravenous injections are available.

Novobiocin. ('Albamycin') is particularly useful against staphylococcal infections which are resistant to other antibiotics. It may cause rashes, and has similar properties to kanamycin.

Spiramycin, Oleandomycin. ('Rovamycin' 'Sigmamycin', which also contains tetracycline.) These have properties similar to erythromycin.

Fusidic acid ('Fucidin') is bactericidal towards staphylococci, and is reserved for treatment of infections due to staphylococci which are resistant to other antibiotics. Usual dose: 2 capsules (500 mg) three times a day with meals.

Clindamycin ('Dalacin C') is given orally, being well absorbed. It is effective against staphylococci, streptococci and pneumococci.

Rifampicin ('Rimactane') is a semi-synthetic derivative of the antibiotic rifamycin. It is active against a wide range of Gram-positive and Gram-negative bacteria, mycobacteria (tuberculosis and leprosy) and the trachoma agent. It also inhibits certain pox viruses e.g. variola minor (a strain of smallpox virus) and vaccinia virus) but unfortunately the high concentrations of the drug which would be required to treat these virus diseases in man could not be maintained.

SPECIAL ANTIBIOTICS

There are a number of antibiotics which are occasionally used for special purposes. They tend to be toxic and are therefore limited in their application. They include:

Neomycin is of value in some gastro-intestinal infections and may also be applied locally to the skin and has similar properties to kanamycin.

Bacitracin, an antibiotic derived from bacillus subtilis which has a limited use against streptococci, staphylococci and some other organisms. It may have a toxic effect on the kidneys and is only given by injection in selected cases when other antibiotics have failed (dose 20,000 units, 6 hourly). It may safely be applied locally to infected wounds.

Polymyxin B is effective against *Pseudomonas pyocyanea* and certain other uncommon organisms. It is given in doses of 250,000 units every four to six hours by intramuscular injection. It can be given intrathecally in special cases of meningitis.

Colistin ('Colomycin') resembles Polymyxin B chemically and pharmacologically and is equally toxic. Principal toxic effects are on the nervous system and kidneys.

Gentamycin ('Genticin', 'Cidomycin') and **carbenicillin** ('Pyopen') are active against *Pseudomonas pyocyanea.*

Kanamycin is primarily of value in the treatment of resistant *B. proteus* infections and also in gonococcal infections when the patient is sensitive to penicillin or the organism is resistant. It is a toxic drug and, like streptomycin may cause deafness.

Tyrothricin and **Gramicidin** may be used as local applications.

FUNGICIDES

Nystatin. This is a special antibiotic which has no action on ordinary bacteria but is effective against fungi and yeasts such as *Candida albicans.* It may be applied locally for thrush and pessaries are available for vaginal infections. Doses of 500,000 to 1 million units may be given by mouth for intestinal and general monilia infections especially those following administration of tetracycline.

Griseofulvin is used in the treatment of fungus infections of the skin, including ringworm. The usual dose is 1 G daily, orally. Treatment may be prolonged if the nails are affected.

Amphotericin B is a fungicidal antibiotic used in systemic mycotic infections with *Candida*, *Coccidioides*, *Cryptococcus*, *Blastomyces* and *Histoplasma*. It is very toxic and may cause kidney damage and, therefore must only be used with great caution.

ANTITUBERCULOUS DRUGS

Streptomycin

This is an antibiotic obtained from a soil organism called *Streptomyces griseus.* It is interesting to note that in the process of its manufacture Vitamin B_{12} is formed, a fact which has made the preparation of the latter substance commercially possible.

Although streptomycin is used mainly in the treatment of tuberculosis, it is also active against a number of organisms (especially Gram-negative bacilli, many of which are insensitive to penicillin, e.g. *Escherichia coli*), which accounts for its usefulness in a number of other conditions. These include some types of pneumonia, peritonitis, cholecystitis, infection of the urinary tract and any condition caused by organisms which are shown by bacteriological test to be insensitive to penicillin or the other antibiotics. In these conditions its administration is only continued for a few days. Streptomycin may be combined with penicillin for use in some infections.

Disadvantages

Like other antibiotics it has certain disadvantages which include:

1. Not only the tubercle bacillus but also other organisms rapidly acquire a tolerance to it and permanently resistant strains of micro-organisms are produced which will no longer respond to treatment with it.

2. If prolonged or heavy dosage, which may sometimes appear necessary in tuberculosis, is employed there is a risk of causing serious toxic effects which include damage to the eighth cranial nerve and the symptoms of giddiness, deafness and tinnitus. The risk increases after the age of 40 years. These symptoms may gradually clear up but in some cases are permanent.

3. Persons who handle the drug may become sensitive to it after a few weeks and may develop a dermatitis of the hands, forearm and around the eyes, which is often very intractable to treatment. Rubber gloves should, therefore, always be worn when administering streptomycin.

4. Hypersensitivity reaction in the patient is usually manifested by fever, often accompanied by a rash.

Streptomycin is used in the treatment of all forms of tuberculosis, the dosage and duration of treatment depends on the individual case.

In pulmonary tuberculosis the dose is usually 1·0 gram daily.

In tuberculous meningitis, intrathecal injections of 100 mg in 5 to 10 ml. of distilled water may be given in addition to intramuscular injections.

It is not absorbed when given by mouth but may be given in this way in certain intestinal infections.

Para-amino salicylic acid (PAS)

This drug which is usually prescribed in the form of its sodium salt (**sodium aminosalicylate**), is not an antibiotic in the ordinary sense but it is used in conjunction with streptomycin for two reasons:

1. It has itself an action on the tubercle bacillus.

2. It delays the development of streptomycin resistance.

The usual dose is 12 to 15 grams daily in divided dosage.

It has a bitter taste and may be taken in water with or without flavouring agents, or in cachets.

In some cases the urine of patients taking PAS reduces Benedict's reagent. PAS is detectable in the urine by testing with 'Phenistix' and this is useful if one suspects that a patient is failing to take his prescribed drugs. It may cause nausea, vomiting and diarrhoea. Hypersensitivity reactions are common and are manifested usually by fever and a rash. Liver damage may occur.

Isoniazid

Isonicotinic acid hydrazide (INAH) 'Pycazide', 'Rimifon' etc.

This is a synthetic substance which has a similar action and which may be given with streptomycin.

The average dose is 200 to 300 mg of isoniazid daily in divided doses.

It passes through the meninges into the cerebrospinal fluid and given with streptomycin, is of importance in the treatment of tuberculous meningitis.

'Inapasade' granules contain both PAS and INAH and are a convenient form of administration. The average dose is 2 scoopsful (packets) twice daily.

Because the tubercle bacillus quickly develops resistance to streptomycin, sodium aminosalicylate and isoniazid when they are given separately (but this is delayed when combinations are used), it is usual to give two of the drugs together. The usual scheme is to give all three "standard" drugs together initially. If the tubercle bacilli are found, in the laboratory, to be sensitive to both PAS and INAH, streptomycin is withdrawn, usually after three months. In advanced cases of tuberculosis streptomycin may be given for six months or more.

The total duration of a course of antituberculous treatment is usually about two years.

Thiacetazone, 150 mg orally daily, is often an effective alternative to PAS, for combined therapy with isoniazid, and is cheaper.

Second-line drugs for the treatment of tuberculosis

Certain drugs are reserved for use in cases where the tubercle bacilli are resistant to or the patient is intolerant of standard drugs.

Ethionamide (0·75 to 1 G daily) is a powerful antituberculous drug but may have unpleasant side-effects. **Prothionamide** has less gastro intestinal side-effects and may therefore be preferred.

Pyrazinamide (maximum dose 1·5 G twice daily) is another powerful antituberculous drug. Liver damage is the most important adverse reaction to this drug.

Cycloserine (1 G daily in divided doses) is an antibiotic with a relatively weak action on tubercle bacilli. Side-effects include convulsions and psychotic disturbances.

Ethambutol (25 mg per kg of body weight once daily) is a powerful antituberculous drug. Occasionally it causes retrobulbar neuritis, an inflammation of the optic nerve, which fortunately resolves completely when the drug is discontinued.

Other second-line drugs are **viomycin, kanamycin, capreomycin** and **rifampicin.**

ANTI-LEPROTIC AGENTS

The treatment of leprosy is often difficult and usually protracted; drugs commonly have to be taken continuously for four years. **Dapsone** is the drug which is most used and is given orally in tablet form, commencing with 25 mg once weekly. Acute exacerbations of lepromatous leprosy (lepra reaction) may be induced by dapsone and require treatment with corticosteroids.

DADDS is in the same group of drugs (sulphones) as dapsone but is long-acting and a single intramuscular injection of DADDS suspended in a special oil provides treatment for 75–90 days. **Clofazimine** ('Lamprene'), a phenazine dye, is the drug of choice when leprosy is resistant to sulphones or is in a state of severe and persistent exacerbation.

Other drugs used in leprosy are **thiambutosine, thiacetazone, rifampicin** (a derivative of rifamycin) and some long-acting sulphonamides (e.g. sulphorthomidine).

Note: PAS, INAH, ethionamide thiacetazone, pyrazinamide and ethambutol are not antibiotics but are included in this section for convenience.

CHAPTER 19

Vaccines, Sera and other Biological Products

The preparation and use of vaccines and sera are closely connected with the subject of **Immunity.**

By Immunity is meant the ability of an individual to resist disease, and is dependent on:

(i) The power of leucocytes to destroy bacteria.

(ii) The presence of antibodies in the blood and tissues which kill bacteria or of antitoxins which neutralize their toxins.

Immunity may be:

1. Natural or inborn.

2. Acquired

(*a*) As a result of recovery from infection.

(*b*) Artificially produced:

(i) Actual immunity stimulated by the use of vaccines and toxoids.

(ii) Passive immunity (by the use of serum containing antibodies obtained from other individuals e.g. human immunoglobulin or animals, e.g. horse serum.

VACCINES

Strictly speaking, a vaccine is a suspension of bacteria or viruses which have been killed or rendered harmless. It, therefore, contains the toxins of the organism which, have been rendered innocuous and can no longer produce actual disease in the individual.

The toxins, however, have the power to stimulate the production of antibodies and, in this way, to raise the resistance of the recipient to a particular organism.

The vaccine lymph used in the prevention of small pox differs from most other vaccines since it contains the living organisms which cause cowpox or vaccinia. The immunity produced by its use depends on the fact that the individual vaccinated contracts cowpox, which is a local lesion at the site of innoculation.

The antibodies to cowpox are apparently the same as those to smallpox and, therefore, an immunity to smallpox remains after the local lesion has healed.

In addition to the above types of vaccine containing organisms, preparations can be made of their toxins, specially made in the form of "toxoids".

Generally speaking, viral vaccines are suspensions of living organisms the virulence of which has been so reduced that no active disease can result.

Technique of administration

Most vaccines are given by subcutaneous injection usually over the deltoid muscle. In most instances further injections (boosting doses) are required at intervals appropriate to each vaccine. Some vaccines can be given by mouth, e.g. poliomyelitis, and possibly by nasal spray.

Reactions

The administration of a vaccine may be followed by a reaction which may be either local or general.

(*a*) Local reaction, with pain, swelling and redness at the site of infection within 12 to 24 hours.

(*b*) General reactions. These include a rise in temperature and general lassitude.

Uses. Vaccines are used to produce an immunity which will prevent the individual from contracting the disease or, at least, modify its severity, if the patient subsequently happens to come in contact with the organism concerned. As already indicated the immunity produced only lasts for a limited period, usually from one to several years, after which "boosting" doses are needed.

In recent years, in order to reduce the number of injections required, it has been possible to combine several different organisms or their toxoids in one preparation.

At one time vaccines were used in the actual treatment of certain conditions, e.g. acne and staplytococcal infections (boils) but other methods of treatment (e.g. antibiotics) are now available.

ROUTINE IMMUNIZATION

Vaccination in infancy and childhood, in particular, have been largely responsible for the very marked reduction in the incidence of a number of infectious diseases and their serious results and complications, e.g. whooping cough, measles, smallpox, diphtheria and poliomyelitis and even to their virtual disappearance.

Special time schedules have been worked out in order to give the maximum immunity when the child is most likely to be in contact with or affected by the disease; i.e. infancy, school entry and later in life.

Diphtheria prophylactics

Originally there were several individual preparations e.g. Alum precipitates toxoid (APT).

Purified toxoid, aluminium precipitated (PTAP).

Toxoid–Antitoxin floccules (Dip/Vac/TAF).

The preparation now in use for primary immunization in early childhood is PTAP which is combined with tetanus toxoid and pertussis vaccine, or with tetanus toxoid and poliomyelitis vaccine. As previously indicated these mixed vaccines reduce the number of injections required.

Diphtheria vaccines may cause severe reaction if given to older children and adults for the first time. A preliminary Schick Test is desirable to detect such individuals. TAF is often preferable in such cases.

Tetanus vaccine (toxoid)

It is now usual to combine this with diptheria immunization in childhood, with subsequent boosting doses. If commenced later, 0·5 ml. is given by intramuscular injection followed by 1·0 ml. in six weeks. Further doses are desirable after 1 and 5 years in order to give full protection. If such an immunized individual should happen to sustain a wound likely to be infected with tetanus bacilli a further dose should preferably be given immediately.

A non-immunized person, in such circumstances, may require tetanus antitoxin (serum) and the administration of penicillin or tetracycline.

Pertussis (whooping cough) vaccine

This is usually given in combination with the two vaccines

previously mentioned. It does not always seem to give complete protection but can be expected to modify the severity of the disease.

Poliomyelitis vaccine

Two types of vaccine have been developed.

(a) **Salk-type vaccine** which is given by intramuscular injection, repeated in 6 weeks and again after 6 months.

(b) **Sabin-type vaccine** which has largely replaced the former for routine use because it is given by mouth, e.g. three drops on a piece of sugar repeated after an interval of 6–8 weeks, with a booster dose every 3 years. It can be given at the same time as the diptheria–tetanus–petussis (DPT) vaccine but is avoided during early pregnancy or any intercurrent illness, or diarrhoea. It contains three strains of polio virus.

Measles vaccine

This is a live attenuated viral vaccine, given by intramuscular injection, of recent introduction. If its use became universal the disease might very well disappear in its epidemic form.

It should not be used in the presence of any intercurrent disease such as leukaemia, Hodgkin's disease or in children taking steroids. Reactions may follow the injection but they are usually mild.

Rubella (german measles) vaccine

This is a live attenuated viral vacine given subcutaneously in a dose of 0·5 ml., to girls at the onset of puberty if they have not by then acquired natural infection. About 15 per cent of young married women have no acquired natural immunity. If they are exposed to rubella during the first four months of pregnancy, their babies may be born deformed, blind, deaf, mentally retarded or with cardiac defects. Hence the importance of vaccinating non-immune girls before they embark on having a family.

Smallpox vaccination

Historically this was the first adventure into the realms of disease prevention for it was Edward Jenner in 1780 who made use of the fact that human beings who contracted cowpox—a local lesion usually on the hands—as a result of milking infected cows were immune to smallpox. Vaccinia is an acute infection affecting cows and characterized by a pustular eruption which is confined to the udder and teats. It is considered that the condition is due to the infection by the virus of smallpox, the virulence of which is so modified by its passage through the body of the cow that only a localized lesion results. Rarely, vaccinia lesions spread extensively over the body—a condition known as *generalized vaccinia*. It occurs particularly in children who lack gamma globulin (hypogamma globulinaemia) and may be fatal.

The material used for the purpose of smallpox vaccination is prepared in the following way. A healthy calf is innoculated with the virus of vaccinia. Vesicles of cowpox develop on the udder of the calf. The lymph from these vesicles is collected and mixed with glycerin, which acts as a preservative. The final product, after tests to ensure its freedom from other organisms, is placed in small glass or plastic tubes and is known as glycerinated calf lymph.

Technique. The site of innoculation is cleaned with soap and water. Antiseptics are not used as they might destroy the virus.

The lymph is introduced into the skin either (*a*) by making a superficial scratch with a needle or point of a scalpel, not more than $\frac{1}{2}$ inch (1·5 cm.) long without drawing blood, through a drop of lymph placed on the chosen spot, or (*b*) by means of the multiple pressure technique using a triangular pointed needle which is held almost parallel to the skin. Fifteen to thirty applications of fine pressure are made through the drop of lymph which are sufficient to roughen the skin and to permit the entry of the virus.

The lymph is allowed to dry and may then be covered by a small sterile but not antiseptic, preferably waterproof, dressing.

The following sequence of events takes place at the site of a primary innoculation. On the third day a red papule appears, by the sixth day it has become a vesicle which reaches its maximum development on the eighth day and has a central (unbilicated) depression. By the tenth day a pustule is formed with some surrounding redness of the skin and local tenderness. The axillary glands may also be swollen and tender. Slight fever and malaise may occur. In the course of 2 or 3 days the pustule dries up, leaving a scab which separates by the end of 3 weeks.

In successful revaccination, the process is accelerated and the lesion is smaller unless a long interval has elapsed since the primary vaccination.

Recent successful vaccination produces complete immunity to smallpox in nine days from the time of innoculation. The incubation period of smallpox is approximately fourteen days. It follows, therefore, that an individual vaccinated within three or four days of exposure to smallpox will obtain protection.

Methisazone ('Marboran') has been shown to protect smallpox contacts even if given late in the incubation period. It is a synthetic drug which is given by mouth, adult dose: 6 G. The drug is not of any value in the treatment of the disease itself but is useful in generalized vaccinia.

Complications of smallpox vaccination

(a) **Local sepsis** which should not occur if the subject is in a good state of health and proper cleanliness is observed.

(b) **Auto-innoculation.** The vaccinee may scratch the itching lesion and transfer virus, with his fingers, to other parts of his body. Vaccination lesions then appear at these sites. If the eye happens to be one of these sites, corneal scarring and blindness may result.

(c) **Post-vaccinal encephalitis** or inflammation of the brain occasionally develops especially in children who are vaccinated for the first time between the ages of 3 and 13. It is a very dangerous condition (mortality 30–40 per cent.)

(d) **Generalised vaccinia.** The law no longer demands that vaccination shall be performed on infants before the age of 6 months. In view of the possibility of post-vaccinal encephalitis in older children, if it is to be included in the vaccination schedule, children should be vaccinated during the second year of life.

(e) A generalized erythematous rash due to allergy.

It should be remembered that smallpox vaccination is compulsory under some circumstances, e.g. travel abroad to certain countries, the Forces, etc.

Routine smallpox vaccination is no longer recommended in the U.K. except for doctors, nurses and others who may come in contact with smallpox.

The immunity conferred by this vaccination lasts about three years and revaccination should, therefore, be performed at intervals of this duration, in particular in individuals who are likely to come in contact with the disease. A lesser degree of immunity persists for about seven years.

SPECIAL IMMUNIZATION

There are a number of infections to which immunity may be confined by the use of vaccines, but generally speaking they are only needed by travellers abroad or workers in special trades, or according to individual circumstances.

Tuberculosis vaccine

A preparation known as BCG vaccine (Bacille Calmette–Guerin) consisting of live tubercle bacilli, specially cultured so that they have become non-virulent and unable to cause disease, has been used to produce a degree of immunity to tuberculosis in newborn infants of tuberculous parents, some adolescents and those who work in contact with tuberculosis, e.g. nurses who are found to be Mantoux negative. An intradermal dose of 0·1 ml. produce a small papule which persists for some weeks. Although this does not promise complete protection it does increase the resistance to the infection.

Influenza vaccine

A single dose containing inactivated viruses of types A and B (or variations of them) may be given in the autumn especially when outbreaks of influenza are anticipated. Although not in universal use they are recommended for individuals who suffer from chronic pulmonary and heart disease in particular.

The injection is given subcutaneously; the dose for an adult is 1 ml. and for a child (6–12 years old) it is 0·5 ml. The vaccine should not be administered to anyone who is allergic to eggs, the influenza viruses having been grown in hen's eggs.

Typhoid vaccine

The vaccine generally employed to produce immunity to enteric fever contains killed typhoid bacilli together with the bacilli which cause paratyphoid A and paratyphoid B, in order that it may be effective against all the organisms of the typhoid group. It is sometimes called TAB, and usually contains:

Typhoid bacilli	1000 million.
Paratyphoid A	500 million.
Paratyphoid B	500 million.

in 1 ml. A first dose of 0·5 ml. is followed by a second dose of 1 ml.
after an interval of 28 days. A third dose should be given six to
twelve months after the second. Those frequently exposed to
infection should be revaccinated every twelve months.

A local reaction occurring at the site of injection, consisting of
tenderness, redness and swelling after four hours is common.
General symptoms including pyrexia or malaise lasting twenty-
four hours are quite common. The subject should therefore restrict
activity during this period and avoid alcohol.

A preparation of the toxin of tetanus (tetanus toxoid) may be
included in order to produce immunity to tetanus at the same time
(TABT). The interval between doses should be four to six weeks.
A third dose may be given after six months. Typhoid vaccine may
also be combined with cholera vaccine.

Other vaccines are available and used according to regional
requirements. They include: cholera, yellow fever and plague
vaccines.

Rabies vaccine. This is necessary for workers in quarantine
kennels and when local outbreaks occur.

Anthrax vaccine is desirable for workers in tanneries and similar
occupations handling raw leather and other animal products.

N.B. Details of available vaccines, their dosage and interval requirements
are clearly listed in the British National Formulary and literature is also
supplied by the manufacturers.

TESTS OF IMMUNITY

Although bacterial toxins themselves are too dangerous for
therapeutic use, very dilute solutions are used in order to test the
immunity of individuals to certain diseases.

If a minute dose of toxin is injected into the skin (intradermally)
and the individual has antibodies to that disease circulating in the
blood, the effect of the toxin will be neutralized and there will be
no reaction (negative response).

On the other hand, if the blood is deficient in antibodies, the
toxin will produce local inflammation (redness, swelling, etc.) and
the reaction is said to be positive. In other words, it indicates that
the individual is susceptible to the disease. Examples of this are:

1. The Schick test for diphtheria

A minute dose (0·2 ml.) of diluted diphtheria toxin is injected directly into
the skin of the forearm (intradermally). If the individual has a sufficient

amount of diphtheria antitoxin circulating in the blood, the toxin is neutralized and no reaction takes place.

Such a patient is immune to diphtheria and the test is said to be negative.

On the other hand, if the patient has not sufficient antibodies to diphtheria present, an area of redness 1·5–2·5 cm. (½ to 1 inch) in diameter develops at the site of injection within twenty-four hours and persists for two to three days. This is a positive reaction.

A control injection is made into the other forearm consisting of diphtheria toxin which has been destroyed by heat. This is done in order to make sure that a positive reaction is due to the toxin and not to the protein contained in it, as some individuals are sensitive to the protein alone.

Immunization. Those patients who have been found to be susceptible to diphtheria by means of the Schick test can be rendered immune by injecting one of the diphtheria prophylactics already mentioned. The body is stimulated to produce a supply of antibodies which lasts for several years. Two or more subcutaneous injections are given and immunity develops about six weeks after the last injection has been made. By this means it has been possible to reduce very considerably the incidence of infection among school children and among those nursing diphtheria.

2. The Dick test for scarlet fever

This is a similar test to the above, using the toxin of the scarlet fever streptococcus in place of diphtheria toxin.

Tuberculin tests

The basis of the various tests for tuberculous infection is tuberculin. This is an extract obtained from tubercle bacilli and contains some of their toxins.

3. The Mantoux test

This consists of the intradermal injection of 0·1 ml. of 1 in 10,000 dilution of Old Tuberculin into the forearm. In a positive reacton an area of redness and swelling develops at the site of inoculation within a few hours and reaches its maximum in twenty-four to forty-eight hours. If negative, subsequent tests may be carried out with stronger solutions, i.e. 1 in 1000 and 1 in 100.

This test is interpreted on a different basis from the tests for diphtheria and scarlet fever. Firstly, a distinction must be made between tuberculous infection and tuberculous disease. Sooner or later tubercle bacilli gain entrance to the body of almost every individual, but it is only in a few that active clinical tuberculous disease develops.

A positive reaction means that an individual has been infected by the tubercle bacillus at some time which may or may not have produced evidence of disease. By this infection he has been rendered sensitive or allergic to the toxins of the tubercle bacillus and the positive Mantoux test is an allergic reaction in the skin to the proteins contained in these toxins.

A positive reaction in young children often indicates active tuberculous disease. Except in special circumstances, a negative reaction indicates that there has been no tuberculous infection.

4. The Heaf test

For this test tuberculin purified protein derivative (PPD) is used. A ring of superficial punctures is made in the skin with a special instrument. The punctures are made through a spread-out drop of PPD. The result is judged by the number of papules which develop.

5. Patch tests

These are similar in principle and consist of the application to the surface of the skin of a patch of material saturated with tuberculin. This is left in position for 24 hours. Local redness and swelling indicate a positive reaction.

SERA

The term serum used in therapeutics refers to the blood serum of an animal which has been rendered immune to a disease by means of a vaccine or toxin. Sometimes, also, serum is obtained from a human being who is convalescent from, or has previously had, a particular disease. Such sera, therefore, contain antibodies to the disease which have the power either of neutralizing the toxins or destroying the bacteria which cause the condition. They may be either:

1. Anti-toxic.
2. Anti-bacterial.

Because they contain antibodies "ready made" by another animal and the individual to whom they are given takes no part in the formation of these antibodies, they are described as producing "Passive Immunity".

Unfortunately it is not possible to produce sera which are effective against all organisms. Further, the introduction of chemotherapy and antibiotics have rendered the use of certain sera obsolete, for example, anti-streptococcal serum and meningo-coccus antitoxin.

Among the more important sera are:
Diphtheria antitoxin.
Tetanus antitoxin.
Gas gangrene antitoxin.
Snake anti-sera.

Serum may be used (i) as a prophylactic agent after exposure to infection in order to prevent an attack or to minimize its severity, or (ii) in the treatment of established disease.

Immunity acquired as a result of an infection lasts for a considerable period and often for a lifetime. Active immunity produced by a vaccine may last several years, but passive immunity obtained by the injection of a serum is of short duration which rarely exceeds a few weeks.

Sera may be administered by the subcutaneous, intramuscular, intravenous, intraperitoneal or intrathecal routes. The rate of absorption is most rapid when the intravenous route is used and this method is also of advantage when large doses have to be given. Intramuscular injection produces quicker results than subcutaneous.

Serum sickness. Because serum contains protein which is foreign in character to that of the individual receiving it, allergic reactions are sometimes observed 8 to 12 days after its administration. These consist of pyrexia, joint pains, rashes such as urticaria (wheals), erythema (general redness), etc. This condition is known as serum sickness and may be relieved by injections of adrenaline (1 in 1000), 0·5 ml., and applications of calamine lotion if the rash is irritating. Antihistamine drugs are also given.

Modern methods of preparing serum have, however, reduced the amount of protein present to a minimum and reactions are not so common as formerly.

Anaphylactic shock. This is a severe type of allergic reaction. If a patient has at any time had an injection of horse serum, in any form, great care must be taken if another dose is given, as the individual is rendered over-sensitive to the proteins contained in horse serum. This over-sensitivity takes about ten days to develop and persists for a very long time. Once it has developed a second injection of serum may cause immediate and severe collapse or even sudden death These symptoms are known as anaphylactic shock. Asthmatic patients are often sensitive to the injection of horse serum, and for these reasons, all patients should be asked if they suffer from asthma or if they have previously had serum, before the injection is given.

Treatment consists of hydrocortisone, 100 mg intravenously, adrenaline (1 in

1000) 0·5 ml., subcutaneously and an antihistamine, e.g. chlorpheniramine ('Piriton'), 10 mg intravenously. The foot of the bed should be raised, so that the head is low.

Artificial respiration may be necessary.

Persons known to be sensitive are desensitized by giving a series of small amounts before the main dose, e.g. 0·5 ml., 1 ml., 2 ml., 5 ml. at intervals of 5 minutes.

In cases of diphtheria which have previously had antitoxin, a preliminary intramuscular injection of 1 ml. followed 6 hours later by the full intramuscular dose of serum has been found satisfactory.

Adrenaline should always be at hand in case of emergency.

Diphtheria antitoxin

This may be given subcutaneously, intramuscularly or intravenously. When large doses are used, the latter method is preferable. The dose is ordered in units according to the severity of the case, irrespective of the age of the patient, and may be repeated in 12 to 24 hours, e.g.:

In mild cases and nasal diphtheria	8000 units.
For moderately severe cases	16,000 units.
For severe cases and laryngeal diphtheria	24,000 to 100,000 units.

Tetanus antitoxin

Anti-tetanic serum may be used prophylactically and for the treatment of the disease.

Prophylaxis. If the patient has not been previously immunized the incidence of tetanus may be greatly reduced by giving appropriate doses of antitoxin without delay to all cases of accidental wounds, in particular those contaminated with road dirt. The minimal dose is 1500 units. In extensive and badly contaminated wounds it is repeated in a week.

A preliminary test dose for serum sensitivity of 0·2 ml. should be given first, followed by the remainder in 30 minutes if there is no reaction.

Treatment. Once the disease has developed, the only hope of success is to administer repeated large doses of antitoxin, e.g.

Initial dose:	25,000 to 100,000 units intravenously.
Repeated daily dose:	50,000 units.
Total dosage:	300,000 to 400,000 units.

I

The symptoms of tetanus are caused by the toxins of the germ in the wound spreading up the nerves (or possibly by the blood stream) to the brain and spinal cord. Once they have reached the central nervous system, the toxins become "fixed" in the tissues and are unaffected by antitoxin. The effect of the latter is to neutralize any more toxin manufactured in the wound and to render it harmless before it can reach the central nervous system.

At the same time, the spasms are controlled by sedatives such as pentothal, phenobarbitone, chlorpromazine, bromethol ('Avertin') or paraldehyde, the last two being given per rectum. Muscle relaxants, tracheotomy and mechanical ventilation may be required.

The prevention of tetanus

In view of its high mortality the prevention of tetanus is of great importance and prophylactic measures are essential in most wounds due to trauma, especially in agricultural and garage workers. Individuals may be divided into two main groups:

1. Immune, i.e. those who have received three injections of tetanus vaccine within five years. A subsequent boosting dose will have given a further period of five years immunity.

Procedure: Such casualties only require a further 0·5 ml. of tetanus vaccine intramuscularly.

2. Non-immune, i.e. (*a*) those who have never received a full course of tetanus vaccine or who have not received a boosting dose within five years; (*b*) if more than a week has elapsed since a previous dose of tetanus antitoxin.

Procedure: (i) Provided non-immune patients have never had any type of serum before and have no history of allergic disease, they should be given not less than 1500 units of tetanus antitoxin at once.

(ii) If serum sensitivity is likely to be present, give test dose of 0·2 ml. antitoxin subcutaneously and wait 30 minutes before the remainder of the dose is given.

(iii) In allergic subjects the test dose of antitoxin should be diluted ten times with saline and 0·2 ml. of this mixture given. If no symptoms develop give 0·2 ml. undiluted toxin followed by the full dose in 30 minutes as in (ii). If allergic shock symptoms develop the patient should be kept warm, lying down and given ml. of 1 in 1000 adrenaline intramuscularly. An antihistamine may be required. If shock symptoms have developed wait until these have subsided (6 to 12 hours) before further doses of antitoxin are given.

(iv) Following the administration of antitoxin the patient should be instructed to have a course of tetanus vaccine viz:

> 0·5 ml. of adsorbed tetanus toxoid on the same day as the antitoxin but in the other arm.
>
> 0·5 ml. six to twelve weeks later.
>
> 0·5 ml. six to eighteen months later with subsequent boosting doses at intervals of five years.

It is important that the patient should have a record card indicating the treatment which has been given.

Anti-snake venom serums

These are used in the treatment of snake-bite. Specific and polyvalent antivenins are available. The dose is 20–50 ml. intravenously.

Human immuno-globulin (Gamma globulin)

This is prepared from the pooled serum obtained from a large number of healthy adults which necessarily contains permanent antibodies to some common diseases from which most of them have suffered in childhood or against which they have been immunized.

Under special circumstances serum from adults convalescent from a particular disease or who have been recently immunized will have an even higher content of antibodies to that particular condition. This may be used in the treatment of vaccinia and in previously unvaccinated smallpox contacts.

The main uses of human immuno-globulin are in women who have been exposed to rubella during the first four months of pregnancy, children who are not immune to measles, especially if they are suffering from some intercurrent disease or likely to cause an epidemic in a hospital ward or institution when they are in contact with other non-immunes. It is also useful in contacts of infectious hepatitis and, possibly, poliomyelitis.

The importance of its use in early pregnancy is the well-known fact that rubella at this stage of pregnancy is very liable to produce congenital deformities in the foetus.

OTHER BIOLOGICAL PRODUCTS

Fibrinogen is available for the treatment of bleeding due to deficiency of this protein (afibrinogenaemia).

Anti-haemophilic globulin (AHG) is available, in short supply, for use in haemophilia.

CHAPTER 20

Radioactive Isotopes

Although not many doctors and nurses will handle these substances personally their increasing use in medicine justifies a brief reference to the subject which, however, cannot be fully understood without extensive knowledge of atomic physics. Nevertheless some of the more simple aspects can be generally appreciated.

1. Basically, matter consists of a number of individual elements alone or in combination.

2. Elements consist of atoms.

3. An atom consists of a central nucleus with a number of electrons revolving round it.

4. The nucleus of an atom consists of two types of particles, (a) protons, (b) neutrons.

5. The number of protons in the nucleus of an atom equals the number of electrons which revolve round it.

6. The chemical properties and characteristics of each element are determined by the number of electrons in its atom.

7. Under certain circumstances the number of neutrons in the atom of an element may be varied. Although the element will then have the same general chemical characteristics its atom will be unstable and it will emit radiation of particles and rays, i.e. it becomes a radioactive isotope of the element.

8. Certain elements e.g. uranium and radium occur in a natural state as a mixture of normal atoms and their radioactive isotopes. Radioactive isotopes of other elements can be produced by subjecting the normal atom of that element to the action of a nuclear reactor.

9. In some instances the isotopes are very unstable and have a short life, that is, after emitting their radiation at a rapid rate the atoms soon return to normal. In others, this process may take days, weeks or many years before the radioactivity ceases, although in fact it is diminishing at a steady rate all the time. This loss of activity is described in terms of "half-life". For example radio-

active iodine (^{131}I) has a "half-life" of 8 days which means that at the end of each eight-day period only half of the radioactivity present at the commencement of that period remains.

10. Radioactivity can be detected and measured by special apparatus, (*a*) Geiger counter, (*b*) scintillation counter.

11. Living cells cannot distinguish between the normal element and the radioactive isotope. If, therefore, a tissue takes up the isotope its presence can be detected and measured by a "counter".

These facts are applied to medicine in the following ways:

1. Research and diagnosis.   2. Therapy.

A great deal of information has been obtained by isotope research on the metabolism and distribution of various substances throughout the body, e.g. the absorption of iodine, its concentration in the thyroid gland and use in the formation of thyroxine. Subsequently, the release and distribution of radioactive thyroxine into the blood stream has been demonstrated.

Although deep X-rays and radium remain the most useful and generally employed methods of radiation therapy for appropriate conditions, radioactive isotopes may be used in certain circumstances, e.g. malignant tumours of the tongue and bladder which were formerly treated by implanting radium needles may now be dealt with by using smaller needles or wires containing isotopes which are more easily handled. Liquid solutions can also be used, e.g. radioactive gold (^{198}Au) solution may be introduced into the pleural cavity in certain cases of malignant pleural effusion or into the peritoneal cavity in some cases of malignant ascites.

Other radioactive isotopes in use are:

(*a*) ^{131}I which given orally in appropriate dosage is an effective method of treating some cases of thyrotoxicosis and a small number of cases of thyroid carcinoma.

Possible risks of ^{131}I therapy in patients with thyrotoxicosis are the induction of thyroid carcinoma or leukaemia. Fortunately these risks appear to be entirely theoretical but, nevertheless, it is recommended that the treatment is reserved for patients over forty years of age. Even then, for fear of genetic effects, it is withheld from women who are or might become pregnant.

A considerable proportion of patients treated with ^{131}I develop hypothyroidism. This requires treatment with thyroxine, usually 0·2 mg/daily, which imposes no hardship.

(*b*) Radioactive phosphorus (^{32}P) is used in the treatment of polycythaemia vera, a condition in which there is an excess of red blood corpuscles. This substance acts by depressing the overactive bone marrow.

(c) ^{131}I and ^{32}P may be used for the treatment of malignant metastases in lymph nodes. The radioactive element, in an oily medium, is introduced into one of the lymphatic vessels which drain into the affected lymph nodes.

The use of isotopes in hospital

All forms of radioactivity, except in the most carefully controlled and minute doses, may affect health adversely. An individual who has been given a radioactive isotope will continue to excrete this in the urine and faeces for some time. The radiation from these excreta might be dangerous to others, especially children and pregnant women, who come in contact with them. Special precautions are, therefore, necessary. A specially screened storage room is essential. All urine, etc. must be collected and stored for several days or even weeks until the radioactivity has decayed sufficiently for it to be disposed of in the normal sewage system. Similar precautions are necessary for any contaminated bedding or clothing.

A hospital unit handling these substances will have special rules and provided they are strictly followed by the staff and patients, the administration of these substances is quite simple and will probably play an increasingly important part in the therapy of the future.

CHAPTER 21

Weights, Measures, Prescriptions and Miscellaneous Tables

The English systems of weights and measures are complicated. In addition to the Imperial or avoirdupois measures used in everyday life, there is a system of Apothecaries' weights which was employed exclusively in dispensing but is no longer lawful.

THE METRIC SYSTEM

The Metric System is used on the Continent and is also being employed increasingly in the United States. It is now being progressively introduced into this country and every new drug is ordered by weight in grams or milligrams, and by fluid measure in millilitres (cubic centimetres and millilitres may be regarded as identical in volume). The nurse must, therefore, be familiar with these measures and should be able to convert doses ordered in Apothecaries' Measure into the Metric System, and vice versa.

Metric weight

The unit of weight is one gram, which is the weight of one millilitre of water.

1 microgram	= 1 millionth part of 1 gram	
1000 microgram	= 1 milligram = $\frac{1}{60}$ grain	
10 milligrams	= 1 centigram = $\frac{1}{6}$ grain	
10 centigrams	= 1 decigram = 1·5 grains	
10 decigrams	= 1 gram = 100 centigrams = 15 grains	
1000 grams	= 1 kilogram = 2·2 (2¼) pounds	

Metric volume

1 millilitre (ml.) = 1 cubic centimetre (c.c.) or 15 minims approx.
1000 millilitres = 1 litre = 1·75 (1¾) pints = 35 fluid ounces.

Metric length

The standard measure of length is the metre (about 39 inches).
  1 centimetre = $\frac{1}{100}$ part of a metre (0·01 metre).
  1 millimetre = $\frac{1}{10}$ part of a centimetre (0·001 metre).

Measures of length, area and volume

1 inch = 2·54 cm.
12 inches, 1 foot = 0·3 metre.
36 inches, 1 yard = 0·91 metre.
16·5 feet = 5·0 metres.
1 sq. inch = 6·45 sq. cm.
1 sq. foot = 0·09 sq. metre.
1 cu. inch = 1·64 cu. cm.
1 cu. foot = 0·03 cu. metre.

Approximate equivalents

The following are the approximate equivalents used in dispensing. (B.P.1963)

Grains	Milligrams	Grains	Milligrams
15	1000 (1G)	1/10	6
12	800	1/12	5
10	600	1/25	2·5
10	300	1/60	1
5	300	1/120	0·5
1	60	1/150	0·4
1/2	30	1/200	0·3
1/3	20	1/300	0·2
1/4	15	1/600	0·1
1/6	10		

Minims	Millilitres	Fluid ounce	Millilitres
5	0·3	1/2	15
15	1	1	30
60	4	20 (1 pint)	600

Conversion of Metric and Imperial Weights, etc.

The most important approximate figures are: To convert:

Weight

grains to grams   × 0·065
grams to grains   × 15
grams to ounces   × 0·03
kilograms to pounds   × 2·2

Fluid

millilitres (c.c.) to minims × 15
minims to millilitres   × 0·06
pints to litres   × 0·57

Domestic measures

1 teaspoonful is just over 60 minims or 4 to 5 ml.
1 dessertspoonful is about 120 minims or 8 ml.
1 tablespoonful is about half a fluid ounce or 15 ml.
1 tumblerful is just over half a pint.

These measures are very inaccurate and should not normally be used.

N.B. A standard 5 ml. spoon is now issued to patients and the unit dose of tinctures and paediatric mixtures has been adjusted to this. Adult mixture doses are 10 ml.

U.S.A. Liquid Measure

The minim, fluid drachm and fluid ounce of the British (Imperial) measure are slightly smaller than the corresponding measures in the U.S. Apothecaries' Measure, but 16 ounces = 1 pint in U.S. measure instead of 20 ounces = 1 pint in Imperial, and therefore the British (Imperial) pint, quart and gallon are considerably larger than the corresponding U.S. measures.

To convert U.S. minims, fluid drachms or fluid ounces into British (Imperial) measure, multiply by 1·0406. To convert the British measure into U.S. measure, multiply by 0·9609.

To convert U.S. pints, quarts or gallons into British (Imperial) measure, multiply by 0·8325. To convert the British measure into U.S. measure, multiply by 1·2011.

WEIGHTS AND MEASURES

Apothecaries weight
(Formerly used in dispensing)

20 grains   = 1 scruple (℈)
3 scruples = 1 drachm (ʒi) =   60 grains
8 drachms   = 1 ounce (℥i) = 480 grains
12 ounces   = 1 pound   = 5760 grains

Care must be taken to distinguish these from the domestic avoirdupois weights and from fluid measures.

Avoirdupois weight

16 drachms = 1 ounce (oz.) =   437 grains = 28·35 G.
16 ounces   = 1 pound   = 7000 grains = 0·45 Kg.
14 pounds   = 1 stone   = 6·5 kilograms

Apothecaries fluid measure

60 minims	= 1 fluid drachm	=	4 ml. (approx.)
8 fluid drachms	= 1 fluid ounce	=	30 ml. (approx.)
20 fluid ounces	= 1 pint	=	0·57 litre
2 pints	= 1 quart	=	1·13 litre
4 quarts	= 1 gallon	=	4·54 litres

Thermometric equivalents

°C	°F	°C	°F
0·0	32·0	38·8	101·84
15·5	60·0	39·0	102·20
18·5	65·0	39·2	102·56
35·0	95·0	39·4	102·92
36·0	96·80	39·6	103·28
36·2	97·16	39·8	103·64
36·4	97·52	40·0	104·0
36·6	97·88	40·2	104·36
36·8	98·24	40·4	104·72
37·0	98·60	40·6	105·08
37·2	98·96	40·8	105·44
37·4	99·32	41·0	105·80
37·6	99·68	42·0	107·60
37·8	100·04	43·0	109·40
38·0	100·40	44·0	111·20
38·2	100·76	49·0	120·0
38·4	101·12	100·0	212·0
38·8	101·84		

To convert °C to °F multiply by $\frac{9}{5}$ and add 32.
E.g. $37°C \times \frac{9}{5} = 66·6 + 32 = 98·6°F$.

To convert °F to °C subtract 32 and multiply by $\frac{5}{9}$.
E.g. $100°F—32 = 68 \times \frac{5}{9} = 37·7°C$.

SOLUTIONS

The nurse is sometimes called upon to make up solutions of a certain strength from other stronger solutions or solid drugs. This practice involves various mathematical calculations in which accuracy is obviously of great importance.

Solutions may be:

1. Hypertonic, isotonic, hypotonic (p. 105).
2. Expressed as a percentage.

3. Expressed (*a*) as grains to an ounce.

                (*b*) as minims or drachms to a pint.

                (*c*) in the Metric System.

4. Saturated solutions.

Saturated solutions

A saturated solution is one which contains as much solid as it is capable of dissolving; any additional amount of solid remains undissolved as a sediment.

It will be clear from experience that some substances (e.g. sodium chloride, common salt) are very soluble and will dissolve in a small amount of water. Others are less soluble,dissolve slowly and require a much greater quantity of water; while some are insoluble.

Further, the rate and degree of solubility is usually increased when the temperature of the water is raised.

Percentage solutions

A percentage solution expresses the number of parts of a drug in one hundred parts of the final solution. The abbreviations "per cent" or "%" are used to denote this. For example:

A 5 per cent solution of dextrose contains:

5 parts of dextrose in 100 parts of the solution
1 part ,,   ,,   ,, 20 ,,   ,, ,, ,,
5 grams   ,,   ,, 100 ml. ,, ,, ,,

Dilution of lotions and other solutions

The strengths of various solutions may be expressed either as a percentage or as 1 part of the substance in a definite volume of the solution, e.g.

        1 in   5 solution = 20 per cent
        1 in 10   ,,   = 10 per cent
        1 in 40   ,,   = 2·5 per cent (2½ per cent)
        1 in 80   ,,   = 1·25 per cent
        1 in 100   ,,   = 1 per cent
        1 in 500   ,,   = 0·2 per cent
        1 in 1000   ,,   = 0·1 per cent

THE PRESCRIPTION

A prescription is a formula stating the ingredients of a remedy with directions for its preparation and administration. (The term is derived from the Latin, *prae* = before; *scribo* = I write.)

The modern prescription, although based on the original form illustrated below should be written in English using ordinary numerals. The doses are expressed in the Metric system and each mixture made up to 10 ml. for adults and 5 ml. for children.

The classical prescription consists of a number of parts:

The name of the patient.
The superscription.
The inscription.
The subscription.
The signature.
The name of the prescriber and the date of the prescription.

These terms can best be explained by examining a typical prescription.

William Smith, Esq.

℞. Potassii chloratis . . . . gr. x
Liquoris ferri perchloridi . . m. xv
Glycerini . . . . . m. xxx
Aquam. . . . . . ad ℥ 1
    Fiat mistura.   Mitte ℥ x.
    Signetur ℥ 1, ter die sumenda, post cibos.

29th February, 1900   John Jones, M.D.

Using abbreviations this would also be correctly written as:

William Smith, Esq.

℞. Pot. chlor. . . . . . gr. x
Liq. ferri perchlor. . . . m. xv
Glycer. . . . . . m. xxx
Aq. . . . . . . ad ℥ 1
    F.M.   M. ℥ x
    Sign. ℥ 1, t.d.s., p.c.

29/2/00   John Jones, M.D.

The complete English translation of the above prescription would therefore be:

William Smith, Esq.

Take thou (a direction to the Pharmacist)
of potassium chlorate . . . . . 10 grains
of solution of iron perchloride . . . 15 minims
of glycerin . . . . 30 minims
Put (or add) water up to one ounce
Let a mixture be made.   Send 10 ounces.

Let it be labelled one ounce (two tablespoonfuls) to be taken three times a day, after meals.

29th February, 1900.   John Jones, M.D.

The above prescription can be analysed in the following way.

Name of patient. This is obvious. The address may also be included. It is also permissible to put the patient's name at the end of the prescription.

Superscription. This is a sort of heading in the form of an instruction to the pharmacist. The symbol ℞ is used and is an abbreviation of the Latin, *recipe* = take (thou).

The inscription. This is the prescription proper and is a list of the various ingredients, together with the amount of each. When written in Latin, it is expressed grammatically in the genitive case because it qualifies the amount 10 grains, i.e. 10 grains of potassium chlorate.

The subscription. This is an instruction to the pharmacist. It states the form which the preparation is to take and the amount to be dispensed.

Fiat mistura (F.M.) means "Let a mixture be made."

Mitte ℥ x means "Send 10 ounces."

Fiat pilula would mean "Let a pill be made."

Fiat lotio would mean "Let a lotion be made."

The signature. This does not mean the signature of the prescriber but refers to the directions to be given to the patient. Signetur or Sign. means "Let it be labelled" and the subsequent instructions may be written in Latin, in abbreviated form or in English.

The prescription is completed by the addition of the doctor's name or initials and the date. When drugs controlled by the Dangerous Drugs Act are included, the total amount of the drugs to be supplied must be stated.

Latin phrases and abbreviations commonly used in prescribing

Ana	aa.	of each
Ante cibum (cibos)	a.c.	before food (meals)
Ad libitum	ad lib.	to the amount desired
Aequales	aeq.	equal
Alternis diebus	alt. die.	alternate days (every other day)
Alternis noctibus	alt. noct.	alternate nights
Aqua	aq.	water
Bis die	b.d.	twice a day
Bis in die	b.i.d.	twice a day
Cras mane	c.m.	tomorrow morning
Cras nocte	c.n.	tomorrow night
Cum	c.	with
Ex aqua	ex. aq.	in water
Hac nocte	h.n.	this night
Mitte	m.	send
Nocte et mane	n. et m. (nmque)	night and morning

Omni mane	o.m.	every morning
Omni nocte	o.n.	every night
Parti affectae	p.a.	to the affected part
Post cibum (cibos)	p.c.	after food (meals)
Pro oculis	p.oc.	for the eyes
Pro re nata	p.r.n.	as the occasion arises (to be repeated when required)
Quater in die	q.i.d.	four times a day
Quantum sufficiat	q.s.	a sufficient quantity
Repetatur	rep.	let it be repeated
Semissis	ss. or fs.	half
Si opus sit	s.o.s.	if necessary (a single dose)
Statim	stat.	at once
Ter die sumendum	t.d.s.	to be taken three times a day
Ter on die	t.i.d.	three times a day

LATIN TERMINOLOGY

The fact that Latin is used, not only in connection with the official terminology of drugs but also in Anatomy and other branches of Medical Science, often adds to the difficulties of the student who has no knowledge of the language or its pronunciation. The following notes on the pronunciation usually employed and the grammar involved may be useful.

Pronunciation

Among the main rules for the pronunciation of technical Latin and of English words derived from Latin are:

ae is pronounced "ee" as in spirochaete, mammae (breasts).

oe is pronounced "ee" as in oedema (a very common mistake is to call this "odema"), oesophagus, oestrin.

-i (at the end of a word) is pronounced "i, long as in like" e.g. ferri (of iron).

-ii (at the end of a word), first "i" short as in tin, second "i" long as in like, as in calcii (of calcium), sodii (of sodium).

c is soft (i.e. like "s") before "e" and "i", as in cerebrum, cinchophenum.

c is hard (i.e. like "k") before "a", "o" and "u", as in calomel, codeina, cum (with).

g s soft (i.e. like "j") before "e" and "i", as in Progestin, genital, gingivitis.

g is hard (as in "go") before "a", "o" and "u", as in gastric, goitre, gumma.

Grammar

The types of word commonly encountered are:

Nouns: names of persons, places or things. In the nominative case (see below) many Latin nouns have the following endings:

-a	e.g.	aqua	-as	e.g.	benzoas
-us		spiritus	-is		cannabis
-um		acidum			

Adjectives: words which express qualities of nouns:

> aqua calida = hot water
> aqua destillata = distilled water

Frequently the Latin adjective has the same ending as the noun as in the examples above, but this is not always so, e.g. injectio hypodermica.

Verbs: words which express an action or state. In the prescription the following are all verbs:

> fiat (mistura) = let (a mixture) be made
> mitte   = send
> recipe   = take (thou)

Prepositions: words denoting the relation of nouns to other words in the sentence:

> per urethram = through or by the urethra

Conjunctions: words connecting nouns or phrases:

et = and (e.g. *Ferri et ammonii citras*—iron and ammonium citrate)
cum = with (e.g. *Hydrargyrum cum creta*, mercury with chalk)

Nouns undergo certain changes in form: Thus there is usually a different ending to denote singular (one person or thing) and plural (more than one).

aqua, water	aquae, waters
acidum, acid	acida, acids
pessus, a pessary	pessi, pessaries
vapor, an inhalation	vapores, inhalations

There is, however, no simple rule which can be given to indicate all the various changes which may occur.

The endings of nouns also change occording to the case. The case of a noun depends on its relation to other words in the phrase or sentence, but the only two of importance in the present connection are the nominative and genitive cases. The former is the subject of the sentence, the latter answers the question "of what or whom". For example, in the description of a drug: sodii sulphas = sulphate (nominative) of sodium (genitive).

It will be recalled that a prescription commences with the symbol ℞ (*recipe*—take thou), the rest of the prescription is therefore written in the genitive case, i.e.

℞	sodii sulphatis
take thou	of sulphate of sodium (both words being in the genitive case, the genitive of sulphas being sulphatis)

ALTERNATIVE NAMES OF SOME DRUGS COMMON

Unofficial or Trade name	B.P. or Official name
Achromycin 240	Tetracycline
Albucid 216	Sulphacetamide
Aldomet 93	Methyldopa
Amytal 139	Amylobarbitone
Anthisan 95	Mepyramine
Antepar 79	Piperazine
Antistin 159	Antazoline
Apresoline 94	Hydrallazine
Argyrol 37	Silver protein (mild)
Artane 156	Benzhexol
Aureomycin 240	Chlortetracycline
Aventyl 152	Nortriptyline
Avomine 63	Promethazine (chlorotheophyllinate)
Benadryl 95	Diphenhydramine
Benemid 194	Probenecid
Benerva 187	Aneurin
Benzedrine 154	Amphetamine
Brufen 222	Ibuprofen
Butazolidine 193	Phenylbutazone
Cardophyllin 118	Aminophylline
Cetavlon 53	Cetrimide
Chloromycetin 239	Chloramphenicol
Chlorthalidone 126	Hygrotory
Choledyl 119	Oxtriphylline (choline theophyllinate)
Cidomycin 242	Gentamycin
Coramine 90, 112	Nikethamide
Cytamen 99	Cyanocobalamin (Vit. B_{12})
Dexedrine 154	Dextramphetamine
Diamox 127	Acetazolamide
Diazepam 151	Valium
Dindevan 109	Phenindione
Disprin 143	Soluble acetylsalicylic acid
Distaquaine 235	Procaine benzyl penicillin
Doriden 139	Glutethimide
Dramamine 63	Dimenhydrinate
Dromoran 148	Levorphanol
Dulcolax 75	Bisacodyl
Edecrin 126	Ethacrynic acid
Endoxana 102	Cyclophosphamide
Epanutin 155	Phenytoin

Unofficial or Trade name	B.P. or Official name
Equanil 151	Meprobamate
Eserine 168, 215	Physostigmine
Eumydrin 66	Atropine methonitrate
Femergin 157	Ergotamine tartrate
Fersolate 99	Ferrous sulphate
Flaxedil 179	Gallamine
Floxapen 237	Flucloxacillin
Fucidin 231	Sodium fusidate
Furadantin 130	Nitrofurantoin
Gantrisin 227	Sulphafurazole
Genticin 242	Gentamycin
Hibitane 41	Chlorhexidine
INAH 244	Isoniazid
Inderal 89	Propanolol
Indocid 222	Indomethacin
Ismalin 93	Guanethidine
Lanoxin 87	Digoxin
Largactil 151	Chlorpromazine
Lasix 126	Frusemide
Lethidrone 112, 146	Nalorphine
Lipiodol 120	Iodized oil
Luminal 155	Phenobarbitone
Marzine 63	Cyclizine
Megimide 112	Bemegride
Mesontoin 155	Methoin
Miltown 151	Meprobamate
Moryl 73, 168	Carbachol
Myanesin 179	Mephenesin
Myleran 102	Busulphan
Myocrisin 221	Aurothiomalate
Mysoline 155	Primidone
Nardil 152	Phenelzine
Nembutal 139	Pentobarbitone
Neo-epinine 118, 167	Isoprenaline
Neo-mercazole 197	Carbimazole
Novocain 159	Procaine
Oblivon 139	Methyl pentynol
Paludrine 219	Proguanil
Pentothal 178	Thiopentone sodium
Phanodorm 139	Cyclobarbitone

Unofficial or Trade name	B.P. or Official name
Phenergan 95	Promethazine
Physeptone 149	Methadone, (Amidone)
Pipanol 156	Benzhexol
Pitocin 206	Oxytocin
Pituitrin 73, 206	Posterior pituitary
Priscol 95	Tolazoline
Prominal 155	Methyl phenobarbitone
Pronestyl 89	Procainamide
Prostigmin 168	Neostigimine
Pycazide 244	Isoniazid
Pyopen 237	Carbenicillin
Rimifon 244	Isoniazid
Salazopyrin 228	Sulphasalazine
Seconal 139	Quinalbarbitone
Serpasil 93	Reserpine
Soneryl 139	Butobarbitone
Sulfasuxidine 228	Succinyl sulphathiazole
Sulfathalidine 228	Phthalyl sulphathiazole
Sulphamezathine 227	Sulphadimidine
Sulphatriad 227	Trisulphonamide
Terramycin 240	Oxytetracycline
Tetracyn 240	Tetracycline
Thephorin 95	Phenindamine
Tofranil 155	Imipramine
Tridione 155	Troxidone
Trilene 175	Trichlorethyline
Urolucosil 228	Sulphamethiazole
Vascardin 92	Sorbide nitrate
Welldorm 141	Dichloralphenazone
Xylocaine 159	Lignocaine
Zyloric 194	Allopirinol

N.B.—Fuller lists are given in The British National Formulary and unofficial publications such as MIMS.

TABLE OF ADULT DOSES

(See also Text)

N.B. I.V. = Intravenous.   I.M. = Intramuscular.
Subcut. = Subcutaneous or hypodermic.

	METRIC up to	IMPERIAL
Acetazolamide ('Diamox') . . .	500 mg	gr. 2 to 4
Acetomenaphthone (Vitamin K) . .	10 mg	gr. $\frac{1}{6}$
Allopurinal	100 mg	——
Amitriptyline	25 mg	——
Ascorbic acid (Vitamin C) . . .	250 g	gr. $1\frac{1}{2}$ to 4
Folic (acid)	5 mg	gr. $\frac{1}{6}$ to $\frac{1}{3}$
Hydrochloric acid (dilute) . . .	4 ml.	m. 5 to 60
Mandelic (acid)	4 grams	gr. 30 to 60
Niconitinic (acid)	100 mg	hr. $\frac{3}{4}$ to $1\frac{1}{2}$
Amylobarbitone (Amytal) . . .	300 mg	gr. $1\frac{1}{2}$ to 5
„ Sodium (Sod. Amytal) .	600 mg	gr. 3 to 10
„ „ (I.V.) . .	1 gram	gr. 5 to 15
Aminophylline (I.V.)	250 mg	——
Ammonium Chloride	4 grams	gr. 5 to 60
Amphetamine Sulph (Benzedrine) .	10 mg	gr. $\frac{1}{12}$ to $\frac{1}{6}$
„ „ (Injection) .	10 mg	gr. $\frac{1}{24}$ to $\frac{1}{6}$
Ampicillin	250 mg	——
Amyl Nitrite (Inhalation) . . .	0·2 ml.	m. 2 to 5
Adrenocorticotrophic Hormone (ACTH) (I.M.)	100 mg	gr. $\frac{5}{12}$ to $\frac{2}{3}$
Aneurine Hydrochloride (Vitamin B₁) .	50 mg	gr. $\frac{1}{80}$ to $\frac{3}{4}$
Apomorphine Hydrochloride . . .	8 mg	gr. $\frac{1}{32}$ to $\frac{1}{8}$
Aqua Chloroformi (Chloroform Water) .	30 ml.	fl. oz. $\frac{1}{2}$ to 1
Aspirin (Acetylsalicylic acid) . .	1 gram	gr. 5 to 15
Atropine: Atropine Sulphate . .	1 mg	gr. $\frac{1}{240}$ to $\frac{1}{60}$
Atropine Methonitrate (Eumydrin) .	2 mg	gr. $\frac{1}{60}$ to $\frac{1}{30}$
Barbitone Sodium (Medinal) . .	600 mg	gr. 5 to 10
Barbitone (Veronal)	600 mg	gr. 5 to 10
Bendrofluazide	2·5 mg	——
Benzhexol . . . (daily)	increased from 2 mg up to 20 mg	
Benzocaine (Anaesthesin) . . .	600 mg	gr. 5 to 10
Bismuth Carbonate	2 grams	gr. 10 to 30
Busulphan	2 mg	——
Butobarbitone ('Soneryl') . . .	120 mg	gr. 1 to 2
Caffeine	300 mg	gr. 2 to 5
Calciferol (Vitamin D) . . .	1·25 mg	(50,000 units)
Calcium gluconate injection (I.M. or I.V.) .	1 grain	gr. 30 to 60
„ Lactate	4 grams	gr. 15 to 60
Carbachol (Moryl)	4 mg	gr. $\frac{1}{64}$ to $\frac{1}{16}$
„ „ (subcutaneous) .	0·5 mg	gr. $\frac{1}{240}$ to $\frac{1}{120}$

	METRIC up to	IMPERIAL
Carbimazole (*therapeutic daily*)	20 to 45 mg	——
,, (*maintenance daily*)	5 to 15 mg	——
Carbon Tetrachloride	4 ml.	m. 30 to 60
Chloral Hydrate	2 grams	gr. 5 to 30
Chlorpromazine (*oral daily*)	up to 800 mg	——
,, (I.M.)	50 mg	——
Chlorambucil	5 mg	——
Chlorothiazide	500 mg	——
Chlorpropamide	250 mg	——
Choline theophyllinate	200 mg	——
Cocaine Hydrochloride	16 mg	gr. $\frac{1}{8}$ to $\frac{1}{4}$
Codeine: Codeine Phosphate	60 mg.	gr. $\frac{1}{6}$ to 1
Colchicine	1 mg	gr. $\frac{1}{120}$ to $\frac{1}{60}$
Cortisone Acetate (*oral or* I.M.)	25 mg	gr. 1 to 5
Cyanocobalamin (Vitamin B$_{12}$)	1000 mg	——
Cyclizine ('Marzine')	50 mg	gr. $\frac{2}{3}$ to $\frac{3}{4}$
Cyclophosphamide	100 mg	
Deoxycortone Acetate (I.M.)	10 mg	gr. $\frac{1}{30}$ to $\frac{1}{6}$
Diamorphine Hydrochloride (Heroin)	5 mg	gr. $\frac{1}{12}-\frac{1}{6}$
Digitalin (amorphous) (German)	60 mg	gr. $\frac{1}{2}$ to 1
,, (crystalline) (French)	1 mg	gr. $\frac{1}{600}$ to $\frac{1}{60}$
Digitalis (powdered) or *Folia* (leaves)	100 mg	gr. $\frac{1}{2}$ to $1\frac{1}{2}$
,, ,, ,, (*single dose*)	600 mg	gr. 3 to 10
Digoxin ('Lanoxin') (*oral, initial dose*)	1·5 mg	gr. $\frac{1}{60}$ to $\frac{1}{40}$
,, ,, (*oral, maintenance*)	0·25 mg	gr. $\frac{1}{240}$
,, ,, (I.V.)	1 mg	gr. $\frac{1}{120}$ to $\frac{1}{60}$
Dimenhydrinate ('Dramamine')	50 mg	gr. $\frac{2}{3}$ to $\frac{3}{4}$
Diphenhydramine ('Benadryl')	100 mg	gr. $\frac{3}{4}$ to $1\frac{1}{2}$
Elixir Cascarae Sagradae	4 ml.	m. 30 to 60
Emetine et Bismuth Iodide	200 mg	gr. 1 to 3
,, Hydrochloride (*emetic*)	10 mg	gr. $\frac{1}{12}$ to $\frac{1}{6}$
,, (*Subcut. or* I.M.)	60 mg	gr. $\frac{1}{2}$ to 1
Ephedrine Hydrochloride	100 mg	gr. $\frac{1}{4}$ to $1\frac{1}{2}$
Ergometrine (I.M.)	1 mg	gr. $\frac{1}{240}$ to $\frac{1}{60}$
Ergometrine (I.V.)	0·5 mg	gr. $\frac{1}{480}$ to $\frac{1}{240}$
Ergotamine Tartrate (*Subcut. or* I.M.)	0·5 mg	gr. $\frac{1}{240}$ to $\frac{1}{120}$
Ethinyloestradiol (*daily*)	0·02 to 0·1 mg	——
Eserine (*see* Physostigmine)		
Ferri et Ammonii Citras	2 grams	gr. 5 to 30
Ferrous sulphate	200 mg	gr. 1 to 5
Glycerin	8 ml.	dr. 1 to 2
Glyceryl Trinitrate (*Sublingual*)	0·5 mg	gr. $\frac{1}{120}$
Guanethidine	10 mg	
Heparin (I.V.)	5000 to 15,000 units	
Histamine Acid Phosphate	1 mg	gr. $\frac{1}{120}$ to $\frac{1}{60}$
Homatropine Hydrobromide	2 mg	gr. $\frac{1}{64}$ to $\frac{1}{32}$
Hyoscine Hydrobromide	0·6 mg	gr. $\frac{1}{200}$ to $\frac{1}{100}$
Imipramine	25 mg	——

	METRIC up to	IMPERIAL
Indigocarmine (*subcutaneous*) . . .	100 mg	gr. $\frac{3}{4}$ to $1\frac{1}{2}$
,, (I.V.)	16 mg	gr. $\frac{1}{8}$ to $\frac{1}{4}$
Injection of Adrenaline (1 in 1000) .	0·5 ml.	m. 2 to 15
,, ,, Calcium Gluconate (I.V. or I.M.)	1·0 gram	m. 150 to 300
,, ,, Mersalyl . .	2 ml.	m. 8 to 30
,, ,, Nikethamide (Coramine).	4 ml.	m. 15 to 60
Insulin		8 to 100 units
Ipanoic acid ('Telepaque') *oral* . .	3 grams	——
Iophendylate ('Myodil') . . .	5 ml.	——
Isoniazid (daily) . . .	200 to 400 mg	——
Isoprenaline (*sublingual*) . .	30 mg	gr. $\frac{1}{6}$ to $\frac{1}{2}$
Kaolin (light)	60 grams	oz. $\frac{1}{2}$ to 2
Magnesium Carbonate (light, heavy) .	4 grams	gr. 10 to 60
,, Sulphate . . .	16 grams	gr. 30 to 240
,, Trisilicate . . .	2 grams	gr. 5 to 30
Meglomine Iodipamide 50% ('Biligrafin') I.V.	20 ml.	——
Mepacrine Hydrochloride ('Atebrin') .	100 grams	gr. $\frac{3}{4}$ to $1\frac{1}{2}$
Meprobamate	400 mg	gr. 6
Mepyramine Maleate ('Anthisan'), daily	300 to 800 mg	
Methadone Hydrochloride ('Physeptone') .	10 mg	gr. $\frac{1}{12}$ to $\frac{1}{8}$
Methylamphetamine ('Methedrine') .	10 mg	gr. $\frac{1}{24}$ to $\frac{1}{6}$
,, (I.M. or I.V.) .	10 mg	gr. $\frac{1}{8}$ to $\frac{1}{2}$
Methyldopa	250 mg	——
Methyltestosterone (daily) . .	50 mg	——
Methylthiouracil . . .	20 mg	gr. $\frac{3}{4}$ to 3
Morphine Hydrochloride . .	20 mg	gr. $\frac{1}{8}$ to $\frac{1}{3}$
,, Sulphate . .	20 mg	gr. $\frac{1}{8}$ to $\frac{1}{3}$
Mucilage of Acacia . . .	16 ml.	dr. 1 to 4
,, Tragacanth . .	16 ml.	dr. 1 to 4
Nalidixic Acid . . .	500 mg	
Nalorphine Hydrochloride (I.V.) .	40 mg	gr. $\frac{1}{8}$ to $\frac{2}{3}$
Neoarsphenamine (I.V.) . .	1 gram	gr. $2\frac{1}{2}$ to 14
Neostigmine (*Subcut. or* I.M.) .	2 mg	gr. $\frac{1}{120}$ to $\frac{1}{30}$
Nicotinamide	50 mg	gr. $\frac{1}{4}$ to 4
Nikethamide ('Coramine') (I.V.) .	2 to 8 ml.	——
Nitrazepam	5 mg	——
Nitrofurantoin ('Furadantin') .	50 to 150 mg	——
oils		
Oestradiol Benzoate (1000 to 50,000 units) .	5 mg	gr. $\frac{1}{600}$ to $\frac{1}{12}$
Oestrone (1000 to 100,000 units) .	10 mg	gr. $\frac{1}{600}$ to $\frac{1}{6}$
Paraffin (Liquid) . . .	30 ml.	fl. oz. $\frac{1}{4}$ to 1
Paraldehyde	8 ml.	dr. $\frac{1}{2}$ to 2
Penicillin (200,000 to 2,000,000 units) .		
Penicillin V	250 mg	——
Pentobarbitone Soluble ('Nembutal') .	200 mg	gr. $1\frac{1}{2}$ to 3
Pethidine Hydrochloride . .	100 mg	gr. $\frac{1}{2}$ to $1\frac{1}{2}$
Phenformin	50 mg	——
Phenobarbitone ('Luminal') .	120 mg	gr. $\frac{1}{2}$ to 2

	METRIC up to	IMPERIAL
Phenobarbitone Sodium (I.M. or I.V.)	200 mg	gr. 1 to 3
Phenolphthalein	300 mg	gr. 1 to 5
Phenylbutazone ('Butazolidine') *daily*	200 to 400 mg ——	
Phenytoin Sodium ('Epanutin')	100 mg	gr. $\frac{3}{4}$ to $1\frac{1}{2}$
Pholedrine Sulphate	20 mg	gr. $\frac{1}{6}$ to $\frac{1}{3}$
Physeptone ('Amidone')	10 mg	gr. $\frac{1}{12}$ to $\frac{1}{6}$
Physostigmine Sulphate	1·2 mg	tr. $\frac{1}{100}$ to $\frac{1}{50}$
Pilocarpine Nitrate	12 mg	gr. $\frac{1}{20}$ to $\frac{1}{5}$
Potassium Bicarbonate	2 grams	gr. 15 to 30
„ Bromide	2 grams	gr. 5 to 30
„ Citrate	4 grams	gr. 15 to 60
„ Iodide	2 grams	gr. 5 to 30
Prednisone	5 mg	——
Primaquine (base)	15 mg	——
Primidone	250 mg	——
Procaine Hydrochloride	120 mg	gr. $\frac{1}{2}$ to 2
„ „ (*subcutaneously*)	1 gram	up to gr. 15
„ „ (*intrathecally*)	150 mg	up to gr. $2\frac{1}{2}$
Progesterone (1 to 5 units)	5 mg	gr. $\frac{1}{50}$ to $\frac{1}{12}$
Proguanil ('Paludrine') daily	400 mg	gr. $1\frac{1}{2}$ to 6
Propantheline ('Probanthine')	15–30 mg	——
Propyliodone ('Dionosil') for Bronchoscopy	16 ml.	——
Propylthiouracil	50 mg	——
Pulvis Ipecacuanhae et Opii (Dover's)	600 mg	gr. 5 to 10
„ Rhei Comp.	4 grams	gr. 10 to 60
Riboflavine	10 mg	gr. $\frac{1}{60}$ to $\frac{1}{6}$
Quinalbarbitone Sodium (Seconal Sod.)	200 mg	gr. $\frac{3}{4}$ to 3
Quinidine Sulphate	200 mg	gr. 1 to 5
Quinine Sulphate	600 mg.	gr. 1 to 10
Saccharin Soluble	120 mg	gr. $\frac{1}{2}$ to 2
Santonin	200 mg.	gr. 1 to 3
Scopolamine (*see* Hyoscine)		
Sodium Bicarbonate	4 grams	gr. 15 to 60
„ Bromide	2 grams	gr. 5 to 30
„ Citrate	4 grams	gr. 15 to 60
„ Diatrizoate 45% ('Hypaque') I.V.	30 ml.	——
„ Iodide	2 grams	gr. 5 to 30
„ Ipodate ('Biloptin') oral	3 grams	——
„ Phosphate	16 grams	gr. 30 to 240
„ „ (Acid)	4 grams	gr. 30 to 60
„ Salicylate	2 grams	gr. 10 to 30
„ Sulphate	16 grams	gr. 30 to 240
„ Thiosulphate (I.V.)	25 gram	gr. 5 to 15
Spironolactone	25 mg	——
Stibophen (Fouadin) (I.V.)	300 mg	gr. $1\frac{1}{2}$ to 5
Stilboestrol	2 mg	gr. $\frac{1}{120}$ to $\frac{1}{30}$
Strophanthin (I.M. or I.V.)	1 mg	gr. $\frac{1}{240}$ to $\frac{1}{60}$
„ G (Ouabain)	0·5 mg	gr. $\frac{1}{500}$ to $\frac{1}{120}$

	METRIC up to	IMPERIAL
Sulphadiazine	2 grams	gr. 8 to 30
Sulphathiazole	2 grams	gr. 8 to 30
Sulphaguanidine	2 grams	gr. 8 to 30
Tetracycline	250 mg	——
Thyroxine	0·2 mg	——
Tolazoline ('Priscol') . . .	50 mg	gr. $\frac{2}{8}$ to $\frac{3}{4}$
Troxidone ('Tridione') . . .	300 mg	gr. $1\frac{1}{2}$ to 6
Tryparsamide (*subcutaneously*, I.M.) .	2 grams	gr. 15 to 30
Urea	16 grams	gr. 15 to 240
Urethane	2 grams	gr. 15 to 30
Zinc Sulphate	200 mg	gr. 1 to 3
„ „ (*emetic*) . . .	2 grams	gr. 10 to 30

Index